What Others are Saying

"Congratulations for your excellent diet guide for Dialysis Patients. You have obviously researched the subject very well. I have reviewed your book and found it to be concisely written and easy to follow. Most published diets can be difficult to understand or follow, and the renal diet in particular can be very daunting and intimidating. I believe your book will be a very valuable reference for dialysis patients and their care givers, as well as for any health care provider involved in the care of these patients. As you are aware, currently available diet guides for this population are extremely cumbersome; they are not so much guides intended for renal patients or their care givers as they are references for dietitians and nutritionists. Your book fills a very important need for a population which unfortunately is expected to increase significantly in the next few years. I will wholeheartedly recommend this book to my renal patients as well as to my colleagues."

David Mayer, M.D.

"The updated publication of *Dialysis Diet* by Judy Mitzimberg remains an important addition to the current resources of educational materials for dialysis patients and their families. Nutrient content of the book is very good, as it contains both potassium and phosphorus, items that are seldom available to patients on food labels. The updated version provides many practical tools to assist patients and families meet their needs without feeling the diet is taking over their whole life."

Elaine Drees MS RD
CRN-NKF Patient and Public Education Committee Chair
Region V Representative

"I found your book very very informative and would actually recommend it to my patients and to the dialysis community. You have done an excellent job putting all the material together and in a format easily understood by the everyday person."

Terry M. Smith, Adm., RN

"This book is very informative with many of the basics of the renal diet. The nutrient content of the book is fairly extensive and it is a great place for patients to be able to learn about foods and nutrient breakdown as it applies to the renal diet."

Debbie Benner, MA RD CSR
CRN-NKF Patient and Public Education Committee

"The *Dialysis Diet* book is easy to read and has invaluable information for those people who are just getting started on the dialysis diet or their care givers. There is information in this book that I would have loved to have had available to us when we were dealing with this issue. It will help to prepare meals with more variety and taste. This is a practical, down to earth book that is written for people who are thrown into this situation with little time to prepare and have limited resources available."

Linda Connolly, LPN
and Daughter of a Dialysis Patient

"Ms. Mitzimberg, you have an invaluable book that to my knowledge, is unique in its form and price. You are to be congratulated for this achievement. I will be sharing this with my patients.

Brad McElwee, MS RD

"I did receive your book and I am using it as an example for my new patients that I educate. I like the simplicity of your presentation as I feel most patients can understand it. I also feel that our patients relate, in a big way, to others wo have walked in their shoes."

Karen Lucero, RD

"Dialysis Diet is an easy to read, easy to reference guide that makes it an excellent meal preparation tool for renal patients and their care givers. Ms. Mitzimberg's book takes information directly from the USDA nutrient database and converts it into a simple, quick, reference guide for everyday people."

Kiki Watson-Scruggs
Client Services Specialist
Niche Pharmaceuticals, Inc.

DIALYSIS DIET

QUICK REFERENCE FOOD VALUE CHARTS
To Assist the Dialysis Patient
in Monitoring

PROTEIN
SODIUM
POTASSIUM
AND
PHOSPHORUS
IN THE DIET

Judy Mitzimberg

ADL Publishing - Glendale, Arizona

All rights reserved. No part of this book may be reproduced or transmitted in any form or by any means, electronic or mechanical, including photocopying, recording, or by any information storage and retrieval system, without written permission from the author, except for the inclusion of brief quotations in a review.

Copyright - 2003

Published by:

ADL Publishing Company
P.O. Box 2791
Glendale, AZ 85311-2791

Cover design by: Christy Moeller-Masel
Edited by: John A. Dahlberg

Library of Congress Control Number: 2002091382

Publisher's Cataloging-in-Publication
(Provided by Quality Books, Inc.)

Mitzimberg, Judy
  Dialysis diet : quick reference food value charts to assist the dialysis patient in monitoring protein, sodium, potassium, and phosphorus in the diet / Judy Mitzimberg. — Rev. ed.
  p. cm.
  LCCN 2002091382
  ISBN 0-9719997-5-9

  1. Chronic renal failure--Diet therapy--Popular works. 2. Hemodialysis--Popular works. I. Title.

RC918.R4M58 2003   616.6'140654
                      QB103-200172

Printed and bound in the U.S.A.

*Written in memory of my Mom,
who lost her battle with
end-stage renal disease on
October 20, 1999.*

Table of Contents

Acknowledgments	i
About the Author	iii
Disclaimer	iv
Note from the Author	v
Introduction	1

Part 1 Helpful Tips

Abbreviations	6
Measurements	7
Protein	8
Sodium	10
Monitoring Fluid Intake	11
Potassium	13
Soaking Vegetables	14
High, Medium and Low Potassium Foods	16
Phosphorus	20
High Phosphorus Foods	22
Eating Enough Calories	23
Tips for Improving Taste of Food	24
Seasoning Guide	25
Nausea and Vomiting	35
Relief of Constipation	37
7 Day Meal Plan	40
Grocery List	47
Dining Out	52
Emergency Diet Plan	81
Vascular Access Site Care	90

Part 2   Food Values

    Introduction   92

To Be Completed by Dietitian
    Daily Allowances   93
    Daily Food Guide   94
    Beverages   96
    Breads   100
    Candy   107
    Cereals   110
    Cheese and Dairy   117
    Desserts   124
    Eggs   133
    Entrees - Frozen or Homemade   134
    Fast Foods   135
    Fish   140
    Fruits   145
    Juices   153
    Meats   156
    Miscellaneous Items   162
    Nuts and Seeds   169
    Pasta, Rice, and Beans   172
    Poultry   174
    Salad Dressings   177
    Sauces and Gravies   179
    Snacks   180
    Soups   183
    Vegetables   186
    Resources   200

Acknowledgments

The revision of this book is due to the responses I received from mailing the original book to various kidney related organizations and dialysis centers across the United States. I want to thank all of the renal dietitians who took the time to review the book and returned positive feedback in their evaluations. Their suggestions for changes and additions are included in this revised edition which makes it a much better resource for hemodialysis patients and their caregivers.

Data Sources:

There are many people and organizations which were instrumental in giving me a helping hand in getting this book to completion.

The phrase "People Like Us" is modified material from copyrighted material titled "People Like Us," specifically the booklet called "Coping" and is adapted with permission of Amgen, Inc. The "Emergency Diet Plan" is reprinted with permission from the Northwest Kidney Centers. The text describing the product Unifiber is taken from a Niche Pharmaceuticals, Inc. letter to pharmacists and is reproduced with the permission of Niche Pharmaceuticals, Inc. and the section "Dining Out With Confidence" is reprinted with permission from "Dining out with Confidence: A Guide for Patients and their Families," ©National Kidney Foundation, Inc. The nutrient values included in the book have been obtained from, and reproduced with the permission of, the U.S. Department of Agriculture from the USDA Nutrient Database for Standard Reference, Release 14.

About the Author

I fell into the field of renal diet planning out of necessity, not from years of study in the field of nutrition.

When my mother developed kidney disease, one of my duties as care giver was the meal planning. As anyone who is a dialysis patient or is the care giver of a dialysis patient knows, this is a very time consuming task. Foods are not labeled to give you the nutritional information you need to monitor the protein, sodium, potassium, and phosphorus that is so critical in the dialysis diet. Balancing each day's meals requires a lot of research.

Through my hands-on experience of caring for my mother and planning all of her meals while she was on dialysis, along with my extensive research since she lost her battle with kidney disease, I came to write and offer this book to you as an aid in the task of meal planning for the dialysis patient in your family.

It is my hope that having all of the information needed to monitor the nutrients in the diet in one place, your task might be a little easier.

Disclaimer

This book is designed to provide accurate information in regard to the subject matter of the book. It is marketed with the understanding that the author is not engaged in rendering medical or any other professional service. The information in no way is intended to be a substitute for dietary guidelines set by your personal physician and dietitian.

Note From the Author

It has come to my attention that the licensing laws regarding end-stage renal disease facilities, as well as the training requirements for dialysis technicians, vary from state to state. I recommend that you thoroughly investigate the dialysis center that you are using or intend to use, just as you would thoroughly investigate any other facility of such importance, like a nursing home. Begin by contacting your state health department officials who oversee this industry; ask them about the training and facility requirements, who oversees the licensing, and how diligent that process is. Next, visit the facilities you are considering; look them over, talk to the staff, talk to the patients; check on the staffing ratio of RNs and technicians to patients; even check on any complaints they may have against them.

Your health and well being is the most important factor to consider, so make certain that you are getting the very best treatment in your area.

Introduction

Who is affected by kidney disease?

People Like Us

As so aptly stated in the People Like Us Family Focus Program of the National Kidney Foundation, Inc., anyone, regardless of who they are, where they live, how old they are, or what type of work they do, can get kidney disease.

According to the National Kidney and Urologic Disease Information Clearinghouse, there are an estimated 245,900 patients on dialysis in the United States. When kidney disease advances to the point where dialysis is necessary, it is called **end-stage renal disease** and requires the patient to have dialysis or a kidney transplant to live.

Judy Mitzimberg

Going on dialysis changes everything about a person's life, but one of the greatest changes is the diet. The nutritional needs of the patient on hemodialysis are different from any other special diet group. The vast majority of the population is programmed to eat heart healthy, low-fat foods, including lots of fruits and vegetables, and to drink at least eight glasses of water a day.

The hemodialysis patient must concentrate on protein and calories while drastically restricting fluid intake. He must eat enough to keep body weight steady when often he has little or no appetite. At the same time, he must monitor the amount of sodium, potassium, and phosphorus in his diet.

Kidney disease is a lot to handle and requires lifestyle changes, not only for the patient but for the entire family. Along with the new routine of being on dialysis, which is very time consuming, the patient and/or the care giver is now faced with the task of planning a diet that will accommodate the nutritional needs of the

Dialysis Diet

patient.

When my mother was diagnosed with end-stage renal disease and was scheduled to begin dialysis, we were provided with some basic guidelines describing the low sodium, low potassium, low phosphorus, low fluid diet that she would be starting immediately. After reading the brochures, it did not sound very complicated. What a shock I was in for.

Sodium, potassium, and phosphorus are found in nearly all foods. The nutrition labels required by the FDA on most food products list the sodium content in the product, but only a few products list the potassium content and I have not found any that list the phosphorus content. Since monitoring of these minerals is so critical to the patient's health and well being, meal planning and preparation becomes a full- time job, almost a new career.

My first idea was to go to the library and get a book on **the renal diet** to answer all of the questions that I had. I went to our local library and to all of the book stores in the city.

There are virtually hundreds of specialty cookbooks dealing with various diets, but I was unable to find even one written specifically for the renal patient. As a last resort, I purchased a copy of *Bowes and Church's Food Values for Portions Commonly Used,* and it became my bible. In the beginning, planning three meals and two snacks each day so my mother did not exceed her intake of the restricted materials, was very time consuming. This is every day, since each and every ingredient in each recipe had to be looked up. It does get easier and less time consuming with time as you become familiar with which foods are high in the restricted minerals.

The amounts of these minerals vary greatly even within the same family of foods. For example, one nectarine contains 288 mg. of potassium while one peach contains only 193 mg. One orange contains 237 mg. of potassium while one half grapefruit contains only 159 mg.

Dialysis Diet

The same is true with vegetables. One cup of broccoli contains 456 mg. of potassium and 92 mg. of phosphorus while one cup of cauliflower contains 176 mg. of potassium and 40 mg. of phosphorus. These are some examples of why you need to have food value charts available when you are planning your meals. Most packaged foods are much too high in sodium for the dialysis diet. It is preferable to make dishes from scratch.

When my mother lost her battle with kidney disease, I tried to think of things that would have made the task easier for me and not so time consuming. That is what prompted me to put together this book of helpful tips and food value charts with all of the information in one place. It is my hope that this will help you understand why these changes in diet are necessary, and also to help make meal planning as simple as possible.

Judy Mitzimberg

Part 1 - <u>Helpful Tips</u>
Abbreviations, Symbols and Measurements

amt	amount
avg	average
c	cup
fl oz	fluid ounce
gal	gallon
g	grams
K	potassium
lb	pound
med	medium
mg	milligrams
Na	sodium
oz	ounce
P	phosphorus
pro	protein
qt	quart
t	teaspoon
T	tablespoon
w/	with
w/o	without

Dialysis Diet

When consulting the food value charts, note that protein is measured in (g) grams while sodium, potassium, and phosphorus are measured in (mg) milligrams.

Measurements

1 t.	1/8 oz.
3 t.	1 T. or 1/2 oz.
2 T.	1 oz.
4 T.	1/4 c. or 2 oz.
8 T.	1/2 c. or 4 oz.
5 1/3 T.	1/3 c.
16 T.	1 c. or 8 oz.
1 c.	8 oz.
2 c.	1 pint or 16 oz.
2 pints	1 quart or 32 oz.
4 quarts	1 gallon
16 oz.	1 pound

Judy Mitzimberg

<u>Protein</u>

Protein has the ability to build and repair body tissue. When your body breaks down the protein, it produces waste products that build up in the blood. These wastes are then pulled out of the body by healthy kidneys or by dialysis, to prevent medical complications.

Once you start dialysis you will need more protein and calories than you did before dialysis. Protein needs to be increased but controlled as well. Too little protein can cause muscle breakdown and increase your chances of infection. Too much protein can cause nausea, vomiting, fatigue, and taste changes.

High quality protein from beef, chicken, fish, eggs, and dairy are better sources than poor quality protein from bread, vegetables, and beans. For your body to utilize the protein for essential functions, you must consume enough calories. It is better to spread your meals out over several small meals during the day instead

Dialysis Diet

of one or two large meals. Your nephrologist and dietitian will determine your personal protein needs and watch your lab values to keep your diet adjusted as needed.

The protein requirement for the hemodialysis patient is 1.2 grams of protein per kilogram of body weight.

Judy Mitzimberg

<u>Sodium</u>

Sodium is a mineral found naturally in almost all foods. Inside the body, sodium acts like a sponge for water. Healthy kidneys keep sodium and water in balance and get rid of the extra sodium and water through urine. This balance helps control your blood pressure. In kidney failure, dialysis must perform this function which makes sodium restriction critical. An excess build up sodium and water in the body causes the body to swell (edema). Your heart must work harder to pump blood with the excess fluid weight, which could result in shortness of breath and/or high blood pressure.

Of all the dietary problems faced by the dialysis patient, controlling the sodium is the most difficult and also the most important. Failure to control the amount of sodium intake will cause excessive weight gain between dialysis treatments, which will make the dialysis more difficult and complicated. Most commercially processed foods are much too high in sodium.

Dialysis Diet

Fresh is best. Learn to use "no salt" or "low sodium" versions of sauces, soups, and vegetables. When buying these specialty products be sure to check the labels carefully to make sure they do not contain potassium chloride.

If you keep your fluid weight gain between dialysis to about two pounds, you should not have to think too much about your sodium intake. If you feel thirsty or if you have gained more than two pounds between dialysis, you have probably consumed too much sodium or fluid. Try to limit yourself to your fluid allowance. Generally speaking, you will be allowed to drink 32 oz. of liquids each day. (This is for a person without any urine output. If you still urinate, your allowance will be higher.

Monitoring Fluid

It is very important to monitor the amount of fluid that you consume to avoid retaining fluid. I found that the easiest way to monitor the fluid intake was to keep a four cup measuring cup next to the sink. Every time I gave my mother anything to drink, either her morning cup of coffee or a small amount of water or juice to take medications, I first placed that amount of liquid in the measuring cup. This way, I could tell when she was getting close to her daily allowance of four cups.

You also have to monitor the liquid for the equivalent of foods that would turn to liquid at room temperature, such as ice cream, ice cubes, jello, etc. Your dietitian can help you estimate the amount of liquid in these foods.

Dialysis Diet

Potassium

Potassium is a mineral also found in nearly all foods and has many functions. It helps regulate the activity of all muscles, including muscles in the intestines, muscles in the heart, and skeletal muscles. It helps your digestion and is also part of the mechanism which helps the body maintain balance between electrical and chemical balances in the body.

Healthy kidneys normally excrete excess potassium from the system but when renal failure occurs, the potassium intake must be strictly monitored. Excess potassium levels in the blood can cause weakness, irregular heartbeat, slow weak pulse, and difficulty breathing.

Because you cannot taste it, potassium is harder to control than sodium in your diet. Do not use salt substitutes as they are usually very high in potassium. The amount of potassium allowed in your daily diet depends on your dialysis and remaining kidney function so always check with your personal physician.

Soaking Vegetables

Many vegetables are high in potassium and are difficult to work into your diet. Soaking vegetables before cooking them will lower the potassium content considerably. This works especially well for potatoes. Use the following guidelines to soak vegetables:

1. Peel and slice the vegetables, then rinse
2. Place the sliced vegetables in a pan of warm water using (5) times more water than vegetables.
   (For 1c. of vegetables use 5 c. of water)
3. Soak the vegetables at least 4 hours or overnight.
4. Drain and rinse the vegetables.
5. Prepare as desired.

Potatoes prepared this way can be used for french fries, mashed potatoes, hash browns, or in soups or stews. They can be stored in the freezer until needed.

Dried beans should be cooked and then soaked. Canned beans can simply be rinsed and soaked.

Soaking removes vitamins from the vegetables as well as the potassium, so consult your personal physician regarding taking a supplement.

Following is a partial list of high, medium and low potassium foods. Most people on hemodialysis may have:

- 1 serving a day from the high group.
- 1 to 2 servings a day from the medium group.
- 2 to 3 servings a day from the low group

Always check with your Renal Dietitian on your daily allowance of fruits and vegetables.

Judy Mitzimberg

High Potassium Foods

Fruits:	**Serving Size**	**K+ Content**
Apricots	3	312 mg.
Banana	1	467 mg.
Dates	1/2 cup	580 mg.
Figs	3	405 mg.
Orange	1	326 mg.
Papaya	1/2 cup	390 mg.
Prunes, dried	5	313 mg.
Raisins	1/2 cup	545 mg.

Juices:		
Grapefruit	1/2 cup	200 mg.
Orange	1/2 cup	248 mg.
Prune	1/2 cup	354 mg.
Tomato	1/2 cup	267 mg.
V-8	1/2 cup	234 mg.

Vegetables:		
Artichoke	1 med.	425 mg.
Beans, kidney, lima, pinto, navy	1/2 cup	350 mg.
Lentils	1/2 cup	365 mg.
Peas, split	1/2 cup	355 mg.

Dialysis Diet

Vegetables:	**Serving Size**	**K+Content**
Potato	1 small	422 mg.
Spinach	1/2 cup	370 mg.
Tomato	1 small	273 mg.
Winter squash	1/2 cup	435 mg.

Medium Potassium Foods

Fruits:

Apple	1	159 mg.
Cherries	10	152 mg.
Grapefruit	1/2	159 mg.
Kiwi	1 med.	252 mg.
Nectarine	1	288 mg.
Peach	1	193 mg.
Pear	1	208 mg.
Plums	2	228 mg.

Juices:

Apple	1/2 cup	150 mg.
Apricot nectar	1/2 cup	143 mg.
Grape	1/2 cup	167 mg.
Pineapple	1/2 cup	168 mg.

Judy Mitzimberg

Vegetables:	**Serving Size**	**K+Content**
Beets, canned	1/2 cup	176 mg.
Broccoli	1/2 cup	228 mg.
Brussel sprouts	1/2 cup	248 mg.
Carrots	1/2 cup	177 mg.
Corn	1 ear	192 mg.
Eggplant	1/2 cup	123 mg.
Peas, fresh	1/2 cup	192 mg.
Peas, canned	1/2 cup	147 mg.
Rutabagas	1/2 cup	277 mg.
Summer squash	1/2 cup	173 mg.

Low Potassium Foods

Fruits:		
Applesauce	1/2 cup	92 mg.
Blackberries	1/2 cup	140 mg.
Blueberries	1/2 cup	69 mg.
Grapes	10	93 mg.
Pears, canned	1/2 cup	119 mg.
Raspberries	1/2 cup	98 mg.
Rhubarb	1/2 cup	115 mg.
Strawberries	1/2 cup	138 mg.
Tangerine	1	132 mg.

Dialysis Diet

Juices:	**Serving Size**	**K+Content**
Cranberry drink	6 oz.	51 mg.
Cranberry juice Cocktail	6 oz.	34 mg.
Hawaiian punch	8 oz.	50 mg.
Lemonade	8 oz.	36 mg.
Peach nectar	8 oz.	100 mg.
Sunny delight	8 oz.	42 mg.
Tang	8 oz.	25 mg.
Vegetables:		
Asparagus	4 spears	96 mg.
Beans, green	1/2 cup	78 mg.
Cabbage	1/2 cup	73 mg.
Cauliflower	1/2 cup	88 mg.
Celery	1 stalk	115 mg.
Cucumber	1/2 cup	88 mg.
Lettuce	1 leaf	19 mg.
Radishes	3	30 mg.
Soaked potatoes	1/2 cup	80 mg.
Turnips	1/2 cup	105 mg.
Water chestnuts	1/2 cup	83 mg.

Judy Mitzimberg

Phosphorus

Phosphorus, like sodium and potassium, also is found in nearly all foods. This mineral is needed along with calcium to build strong bones and teeth, and also to help nerves and muscles work. When kidneys are not functioning properly, phosphorus tends to build up in the blood stream, causing calcium levels to drop. Calcium is then released from the bones into the bloodstream resulting in bones becoming brittle from lack of calcium.

If you find it difficult to limit the amount of dairy products you are using in your diet, there are some things you can do to reduce the amount of phosphorus.

- Take your phosphate binders with meals and snacks.
- Use cream cheese in place of regular cheese on sandwiches and in casseroles.
    2/3 cup cream cheese =
    1 phosphorus serving
- Use sour cream on fruits or in dips in place

Dialysis Diet

of yogurt.

> 1 1/2 cup sour cream =
> 1 phosphorus serving

- Use non-dairy creamer on cereals, in cream style soups, and in puddings and custards.

> 2 cups milk substitute =
> 1 phosphorus serving

If your recipe calls for 1/2 cup milk, mix 2 to 3 tablespoons of dry non-dairy creamer in 1/2 cup of warm water instead, or use 1/2 cup liquid non dairy creamer.

- Limit milk, cheese, dried bean/peas, nuts/seeds, chocolate and liver in your diet.

Name Brand Non-Dairy Creamers

- Borden Cremora - dry
- Carnation Coffee Mate - dry
- Carnation Coffee Mate - liquid, refrigerated
- Coffee Rich - Frozen
- Coffee Rich - liquid, refrigerated
- International Delight - liquid, refrigerated

Judy Mitzimberg

To lower phosphorus levels, the following high phosphorus foods should be limited:

Milk	Cheese
Yogurt	Ice Cream
Pudding	Custard
Cream soups	Casseroles with cheese
Bran	and milk
Bran flakes	Bran muffins
Brown rice	Wheat germ
Raisin bran	100% bran or whole
Navy beans	grain
Kidney beans	Lima beans
Pinto beans	Blackeyed peas
Lentils	Soybeans
Almonds	Cashews
Coconut	Pecans
Walnuts	Peanuts
Peanut butter	Pumpkin seeds
Sunflower seeds	Cola (RC, Coke, Pepsi)
Chocolate	Cocoa
Molasses	Dried fruits
Pizza	Beer
Beef liver	Liver sausage
Liverwurst	Livercheese

Dialysis Diet

Eating Enough Calories

There may be days when you are on dialysis when you just have no appetite. It is not uncommon to experience some loss of appetite due to the fact that foods now taste different. The changes in the taste of certain foods may be caused in part by the medications you are taking and also from the new restrictions in your diet such as the sodium restriction.

It is very important that you eat well to help you feel your best. The following are some things you can try on those days when you aren't feeling hungry to help you eat the necessary amount of calories:

- Check with your Renal Dietitian about starting a nutrition supplement.
- Instead of eating regular meals, try eating smaller meals more often. Eating five or six small meals will help you consume more calories without feeling so full.
- Find out what time of day is easiest for you to eat, then eat your largest meal of

the day at that time.
- Keep snacks on hand that are easy to fix and easy to get to.
- Try increasing your exercise; increased activity often will increase your appetite.

Tips for Improving the Taste of Your Food
- Season or marinade meat, poultry and fish ahead of time with onion, garlic and other herbs mixed with vinegar, lime juice and oil.
- Cook meat, poultry and fish at a lower temperature to preserve natural juices.
- Steam vegetables instead of boiling them.

Discuss with your doctor taking a zinc supplement. Some studies have shown that zinc has some benefit in improving taste disturbances. You can also experiment with new seasonings to enhance the flavor of your food.

Dialysis Diet

Seasoning Guide

Most recipes are high in sodium, but by deleting the salt and substituting various seasonings you can turn them into tasty low-sodium dishes.

The following are some combinations of seasonings to use with various foods. When possible, use fresh seasonings. Sugar enhances the flavor of foods just like salt, so keep a shaker of sugar on the table to use on fresh vegetables. Sugar also can be added to sauces and soups.

Fish:
Breaded/battered fillets: Dry mustard and onion, oregano, basil and garlic, or thyme

Broiled steaks or fillets: Chili or curry powder

Fillets in butter sauce: Thyme and chervil, dill, or fennel.

Fish soup: Italian seasoning, bay leaf, thyme and tarragon

Fish cakes: Tarragon and savory, dry mustard and white pepper, red pepper and oregano

Beef:
Roast beef: Basil and oregano, bay leaf, nutmeg, tarragon and marjoram

Beef stew: Chili powder, bay leaf and tarragon, caraway, marjoram

Meat balls: Garlic and thyme, basil, oregano and onion, black pepper and dry mustard

Swiss steak: Rosemary and black pepper, bay leaf, thyme and clove

Poultry:
Fried chicken: Basil, oregano and garlic, onion and dill, sesame seed and nutmeg

Roast chicken and turkey: Ginger and garlic, onion, thyme and tarragon

Dialysis Diet

Gravies:

Brown gravy: Chervil and onion, onion, bay leaf and thyme, onion and nutmeg, tarragon

Chicken gravy: Dry mustard, ginger and garlic, marjoram, thyme and bay leaf.

Cream gravy: White pepper and dry mustard, curry powder, dill, onion and paprika, tarragon and thyme

Soups:

Chicken soup: Thyme and savory, ginger, clove, white pepper and allspice

Clam chowder: Basil and oregano, nutmeg and white pepper, thyme and garlic powder

Vegetable soup: Italian seasoning, paprika and caraway, rosemary and thyme, fennel and thyme

Salads:

Chicken salad: Curry or chili powder, Italian seasoning, thyme and tarragon

Judy Mitzimberg

Coleslaw: Dill, caraway, poppy, dry mustard and ginger

Macaroni salad: Dill, basil, thyme and oregano, dry mustard and garlic

Potato salad: Chili powder, curry, dry mustard and onion

Pasta and Rice:
Spaghetti: Italian seasoning and nutmeg, oregano, basil and nutmeg, red pepper and tarragon

Spanish rice: Cumin, oregano and basil, Italian seasoning

Vegetables:
Asparagus: Ginger, sesame seed, basil and onion, lemon

Broccoli: Italian seasoning, marjoram and basil, nutmeg and onion, sesame seed, lemon

Dialysis Diet

Carrots: Ginger, nutmeg, onion and dill

Cauliflower: Dry mustard, basil, paprika and onion

Green beans: Onion and dill, parsley, lemon pepper and dry mustard

Squash: Cinnamon, ginger, ground pepper and onion, basil

Beets: Lemon, sugar, vinegar and cloves, dill

There are some seasoning mixes that you can prepare yourself to keep in a shaker on the table and to use while cooking>

All Purpose Seasoning

1 T. Garlic powder   4 T. Basil
4 T. Oregano   4 t. Onion powder
2 t. Marjoram   2 t. Dill weed
2 t. Rosemary   2 t. Sage
1 t. Ground pepper
Blend ingredients and store in a glass shaker.

Judy Mitzimberg

Mexican Seasoning

3 T. Chili powder   1 T. Ground cumin
1 t. Onion powder   1 t. Garlic powder
1/4 t. Ground black pepper

Seafood Seasoning

1 T. Dried crushed chives   1 t. Dried parsley
1/2 t. Ground pepper   1/2 t. Dill weed
1/2 t. Onion powder   1/4 t. Marjoram
1/4 t. Dried lemon peel

Guide to Fresh Herbs

The flavor and aroma of fresh herbs add diversity to your cooking. Since people are more aware of reducing salt and fat in their diets, fresh herbs are now being sold in super markets and at road side farmer's markets. Select just enough to be used, dried, or frozen the same day.

Following is a description of the most popular herbs and some of their uses:

Dialysis Diet

- **Basil -** A commonly used herb that adds a minty, clove like aroma and pungent taste to spaghetti sauce, sandwiches, fish, poultry, squash, cabbage, beans and pasta.
- **Bay Leaf** - A long dull green leaf about 1/2 inch long, this herb is used to season soups, stews, beef, meat marinade, salmon or white fish.
- **Chervil** - Has a sweet taste similar to tarragon. Use it to season soups, stews, fish and steamed vegetables. Add near the end of cooking time in soups and stews and may be used in recipes calling for tarragon.
- **Chives** - Mild onion flavored leaves will enhance almost any recipe. Use liberally on fish, chicken or eggs and with buttered steamed vegetables such as carrots, green beans, sweet corn, squash and cauliflower.
- **Cilantro** - Also known as coriander this herb adds an aromatic sage-citrus flavor to salsas and sauces. A little goes a long way so use sparingly.

- **Dill** - This anise, parsley, celery flavored herb is excellent with poached salmon and fresh buttered steamed vegetables. Dill seed is also a popular seasoning item.
- **Fiddlehead Fern** - This is any fern at the growth stage when it first pokes it's head up through the soil but has not yet begun to uncurl. Select small sprouts, no more that 1/2 inch in diameter. Serve steamed as a side dish.
- **Marjoram** - A strong accenting herb used best with egg dishes, cottage cheese, soups, steamed vegetables or on lamb.
- **Mint** - Sweet flavored with a cool aftertaste. Usually used in desserts but refreshing in summer drinks such as tea, lemonade and punch. It is a fundamental ingredient in lamb dishes and goes well with green salads, carrots, green beans and beets.
- **Parsley** - Most commonly used as a garnish, the snipped leaves add a mild taste to soups, vegetables and sandwiches.

- **Rosemary** - Aromatic, pungent herb usually associated with lamb dishes, it also goes well sprinkled over any roasted meat. Can be used with or in place of basil.
- **Sage** - Gray green leaves with a pebbly surface, sage is a common seasoning in poultry seasoning. It compliments most vegetables but use sparingly as the musty taste can be overpowering.
- **Savory** - This herb is usually used in soups and stews. It has a slightly sharp taste but may be used sparingly on fish, poultry or green beans.
- **Tarragon** - With it's spicy sharp flavor, this herb is excellent for marinades for grilled meats. Also used in mustard and tartar sauce. Should be used sparingly.
- **Thyme** - Used to season meat or poultry stuffing. Has a minty yet lemony aroma and works well to season chicken, vegetables and creole dishes. Rub on meat before roasting to season it.

For herbs that you are not familiar with, try

mixing a small amount with butter or margarine. Let stand for at least one hour then spread on a cracker and taste.

Flavors of herbs are lost through extended cooking. Add to soups or stews approximately 45 minutes before cooking time is complete. For cold foods such as dips they should be added several hours before use or allowed to sit overnight.

To use dried herbs, crush them after measuring to release their flavor. Dried herbs are more intense than fresh. Powdered herbs are stronger that crushed. A good formula is:
1/4 t. powdered = 3/4 to 1 t. crushed
3/4 to 1 t. crushed = 2 t. fresh

Dialysis Diet

Nausea and Vomiting

Sometimes when you first start dialysis, you may experience some nausea and vomiting. This can be caused by several things such as:
1. The rapid change in the body's fluid and chemical balance <u>during</u> treatment.
2. Not enough hemodialysis resulting in uremia. Extra wastes and toxins being left in the body.

This unpleasant side effect of dialysis can usually be relieved by making adjustments to your treatment and diet. Discuss the necessary changes with your nephrologist and dietitian.

If you are experiencing nausea and vomiting, you could notice some weight loss. It is very important to maintain your weight. Some things that may help are:
1. Eat small frequent meals instead of one or two large meals.
2. Eat a cracker or dry toast.
3. Avoid food cooking odors. Usually they only make the nausea worse.

4. Drink as much clear liquid such as 7-Up, broth, water or tea as you are allowed without exceeding your daily allowance of liquids to replace the fluid lost from the vomiting.

Dialysis Diet

Relief of Constipation

Many people on dialysis suffer from constipation. This may be caused by the medications you are taking. Fiber in your diet will help.

Some things you can try to help relieve the problem of constipation are:
- Increase your fiber intake by eating all of the fruits and vegetables planned for you in your daily diet.
- Light exercise; physical activity tends to stimulate the blood circulation in your intestinal tract.
- Drink all the fluids that you are allowed each day.
- Keep regular hours: A regular routine in your life helps to keep your bowel habits routine as well.
- Drink warm water first thing in the morning. Often a warm drink will stimulate the bowels, but keep in mind that this warm drink should be counted as part of your daily allowance of fluids.

Judy Mitzimberg

- Increase fiber slowly. Adding too much too fast may cause problems such as gal bloating and cramps.

My mother's dietitian recommended a product called **Unifiber**, that she used and was very pleased with. Unifiber requires no additional liquids plus it can be mixed with nearly all foods. Unifiber is a totally natural fiber product. Be sure to check with your personal physician before taking any form of laxative.

Try to include some fiber at each meal. Following are some suggestions:

Low-Fiber Foods	**Higher-Fiber Foods**
Instead of...	Try...
Farina	Shredded wheat
White rice	Brown rice
White bread	Whole wheat bread
Low salt potato chips	Popcorn

Dialysis Diet

Lettuce	Cabbage
Green beans	Corn
Bread crumbs in meatloaf	Oatmeal in meatloaf
Plain pasta	Whole wheat pasta . . .
All purpose flour	Whole wheat flour
Apple juice or lemonade	Fresh blueberries or strawberries

Some of these foods may contain more potassium and phosphorus than your diet allows. Discuss with your dietitian about which foods are best for your to try.

Judy Mitzimberg

Seven-day Meal Plan

Below is a seven-day sample menu containing approximately 2000 mg. sodium, 2000 mg. potassium, and 1000 to 1200 mg. phosphorus.

Day 1:
Morning

2 Poached eggs

1 slice Toast w/margarine

2 slices Bacon

1/2 c. Orange juice

1 c. Coffee

Noon

Sandwich

    3 oz. Tuna (rinsed)

    2 T. Mayonnaise

    2 Slices bread

    1 Lettuce leaf

    1/2 c. Pear slices

Evening

Beef Stroganoff - 3 oz. Beef, 1/3 c. sauce

1 c. Noodles

1 slice French bread

1 T. Margarine

Dialysis Diet

1 c. Salad w/oil and vinegar
Snack
2 Graham crackers
Totals:
Na - 1899 mg   K - 1923 mg.   P - 1108 mg.

Day 2:

2 fried Eggs
1 slice Toast w/margarine
1/2 Grapefruit
1 c. Coffee
Noon
Sandwich
> 3 oz. Chicken
> 2 slices Bread
> 2 T. Margarine
> 1 Lettuce leaf

Evening
4 oz. Halibut, baked
1 c. Rice
1/2 c. Broccoli
1 Dinner roll
1 T. Margarine
1/2 c. Vanilla ice cream
Snack

Judy Mitzimberg

1 c. Jello w/whipped toppiing

Totals

Na - 1866 mg   K - 1706 mg.   P - 944 mg.

Day 3:

Morning

1 slice French toast

1 T. Margarine

2 T. Syrup

1/2 c. Cream of Wheat

1/4 c. Half and half

1 T. Sugar or sugar susbstitute

1 c. Coffee

Noon

Sandwich

> 3 oz. Hamburger patty
>
> Hamburger bun
>
> 1 T. Mayonnaise
>
> 1 t. Mustard
>
> 1 Lettuce leaf

1/2 c. Apple juice

Evening

3 oz. Pork chop

1/2 c. (Soaked) Mashed potatoes

1/4 c. Gravy

Dialysis Diet

1/2 c. Green beans
1/2 c. Salad w/Italian dressing
1/2 c. Fruit cocktail
Snack
1 pc. Angel food cake w/whipped topping
Totals
Na - 1920 mg.   K - 1558 mg.   P - 724 mg.

Day 4:
Morning
Mexican Omelet
1 slice Toast w/margarine
1 c. Coffee
Noon
3 oz. Fish fillet, breaded, fried
4 spears Asparagus
1 slice Bread w/margarine
Evening
1 c. Homemade beef stew
1 c. Salad w/vinegar and oil
1 slice Bread w/margarine
1 c. Applesauce
Snack
3 Vanilla wafers
Totals
Na - 1948 mg.   K - 1902 mg.   P - 837 mg.

Day 5:
Morning

2 Scrambled eggs

1/2 English muffin

1 T. Margarine

1 T. Peanut butter

1/2 c. Oatmeal

1/4 c. Half and half

1 T. Sugar or sugar substitute

1 c. Coffee

Noon

1 slice Pizza w/cheese

1 c. Salad w/Italian dressing

1 Tangerine

Evening

1 Stuffed green pepper

1 Dinner roll w/margarine

1 c. Rice pudding made w/non-dairy creamer

Snack

1/2 c. Raspberries w/1 T. sour cream

Totals

Na - 2162 mg.   K - 1754 mg.   P - 1046 mg.

Day 6:
Morning

1/2 c. Cream of Wheat

1/3 c. Half and half

1 T. Sugar or sugar substitute

2 slices Toast w/margarine

1/2 Banana

1 c. Coffee

Noon

1 Tostada w/guacamole

1 Apple

Evening

1 c. Homemade chicken and noodles

1/2 c. Beets

1 c. Salad w/Thousand island dressing

3 Shortbread cookies

Snack

1 Boiled egg w/mayonnaise

Totals

Na - 2093 mg.   K - 2001 mg.   P - 804 mg.

Judy Mitzimberg

Day 7:
Morning

1 slice French toast

1 T. Margarine

2 T. Syrup

2 links Pork sausage

1/2 Banana

1 c. Coffee

Noon

Leftover stuffed green pepper

1 c. Salad w/Italian dressing

10 Grapes

Evening

3 oz. Baked chicken breast

1/2 c. Coleslaw

1 slice Garlic bread

1 slice Cheese cake

Snack

1/2 c. Blueberries w/sour cream

Totals

Na - 1973 mg.   K - 1941 mg.   P - 796 mg.

Dialysis Diet

Grocery List

Following is a list of foods that are okay to eat on the renal diet. This can serve as a starting point for meal planning but does not mean your diet will be restricted to only these foods. Always check with your renal dietitian for your exact diet.

Dairy Products:
Butter
Cream Cheese
Whipped Cream

Non-Dairy Products
Non-Dairy Creamer
Non-Dairy Whipped Topping
Mocha Mix Frozen Desserts
    (Vanilla & Strawberry)
Margarine
Cooking Oils
Mayonnaise
Miracle Whip

Judy Mitzimberg

Meats:

Egg	Chicken
Fish	Lamb
Beef	Pork
Turkey	Tuna
Veal	Chicken livers

Grains and Starches:

Italian Bread	White Rice
French Bread	Noodles and Pasta
Sourdough Bread	Oatmeal
Sandwich Bread	Grits
Croissants	Cream of Wheat
Bagels (plain)	Cream of Rice
English Muffins	Cornflakes
Cornbread	Rice Krispies
Biscuits	Special K
Tortillas	Product 19
Pita Bread	Puffed Rice
Dinner Rolls	Puffed Wheat
	Rice Chex
	Corn Chex

Cakes and Pies:

Pound Cake
Angel Food Cake
White Cake
Lemon Cake
Yellow Cake
Lemon Cremes
Butter Cookies
Sugar Cookies
Vanilla Wafers
Vanilla Cremes

Apple Pie/Danish
Blueberry Pie/
   Danish
Cherry Pie/Danish
Pineapple Pie/
   Danish
Lemon Meringue
   Pie/Danish
Raspberry Pie/
   Danish

Vegetables:

Asparagus
Beets, cooked
Cabbage
Cauliflower
Celery
Carrots, cooked
Corn
Cucumber
Dandelion Greens
   1/2 cup

Fruits:

Apple
Applesauce
Apple juice
Cherries
Canned Peaches
Canned Pears
Canned Fruit
   Cocktail
Cranberries
Cranberry juice

Judy Mitzimberg

Vegetables:

Eggplant
Endive
Escarole
Green Beans
Green Pepper
Lettuce
Mixed Vegetables
Mushrooms
Mustard Greens
  1/2 cup
Okra
Onion
Peas
Peas and Carrots
Radishes
Turnip Greens
  1/2 cup
Wax Beans
Zucchini

Fruits:

Blueberries
Grapefruit half
Grapefruit Juice
Grapes
Grape Juice
Pineapple
Pineapple Juice
Plums
Raspberries
Strawberries
Tangerines

Dialysis Diet

Sweets:	**Seasonings:**
Hard Candy	Basil
Peppermints	Bay Leaf
Lemon Drops	Dill
Sour Balls	Garlic
Red Licorice	Hot Peppers
Gum	Oregano
Marshmallows	Parsley
Koolade	Sage
7-Up	Thyme
Gingerale	Allspice
Soda (not cola)	Cinnamon
Syrups	Cloves
Jams	Lemon
Jellies	Curry Powder
Honey	Ginger
	Nutmeg
	Tabasco Sauce

Judy Mitzimberg

DINING OUT WITH CONFIDENCE

A Guide for Patients with Kidney Disease

**Reprinted with permission from
"Dining Out With Confidence:
A Guide for Patients and Their Families,"
©National Kidney Foundation, Inc.**

Most people enjoy eating out. This guide gives ideas for making your dining experience fun--- even with your special diet. Start by learning your diet well and asking your dietitian for any tips or advice. If you have sodium, potassium phosphorus or protein restrictions, this booklet will help you make good decisions based on your specific diet needs.

Plan ahead

If you will be eating dinner out, plan breakfast and lunch at home accordingly. Cut back on serving sizes and foods high in sodium and potassium during the day. Call ahead to learn more about the menu and how the food is prepared. Explain that you are following a special diet.

Choose a restaurant where it will be easiest to select foods best suited for your diet. Restaurants where food is made to order are the best choice. Restaurant personnel are accustomed to special requests for food items or methods of preparation. However, many require that you call at least 24 hours in advance to make arrangements.

Making your selections

Look over the menu carefully. Ask your server for more detail about items you do not understand. Practice making special requests about the way your food is prepared or served. Consider sharing a main dish with a friend or family member.

Examples of special requests

For salad dressings, gravies or sauces :
"...on the side."
For any grilled, sauteed or baked entrees:
"No salt, please."
For Asian foods: "...with no MSG (monosodium glutamate)."
For sandwiches or burgers: "...without cheese."
"Mustard and catsup on the side."

Protein concerns

If your specific diet includes restriction, you may want to request half portions of main dishes that contain meat, poultry, fish, or cheese. You could share a main dish with a dining companion. Another option is to take part of your main dish home in a doggy bag.

Don't forget that protein is found in cheese and cream sauces; food prepared with milk, nuts and eggs; and in vegetarian dishes containing dried beans or lentils.

Guidelines for specific meals or courses

Breakfast: Breakfast may be one of the easiest meals to eat out. Most restaurants offer a' la carte breakfast items.

Beverages:
Tip: Save your fluids throughout the day to allow more when you are eating out.
- Plan the amount of fluid you may have during the meal.
- Plan when you want the beverage: before, during or after the meal. Decline offers at other times.

Better Choices	Poor Choices
Eggs, cooked to order	Cured or salted meats or fish, such as ham, sausage, lox and Canadian bacon. Limit bacon to 2 strips occasionally
Omelets with low-potassium vegetables such as mushrooms or squash	Omelets with cheese or above meats; fast-food breakfast sandwiches, breakfast burritos
Toast, bagels, English muffins, croissants, plain or blueberry muffins	Biscuits and bran muffins.
Pancakes, waffles, French toast.	Home fries or hash brown potatoes

Dialysis Diet

Better Choices	Poor Choices
Margarine, jelly, honey, cinnamon, sugar and syrup	Real maple syrup or gravy
Low-potassium fruits and juices such as applesauce or apple juice	Fruits and juices such as orange juice or fresh grapefruit half
Hot and cold cereals	Bran cereals and granola with nuts, seeds or wheat germ
Donuts, Danish pastry, sweet rolls, coffee cake	Pastries containing chocolate, nuts, coconut or caramel

- Choose beverages low in potassium and phosphorus. (Ask your dietitian for specific guidelines.)
- Request that your glass or cup not be refilled. Order beverages by the glass instead of ordering a pitcher of drinks.
- Squeeze lemon wedges in your water to help quench your thirst.

- Turn cups or glasses upside down before they are filled, or ask to have them removed.
- Push your glass or cup away from your plate when your are finished to avoid refills.

Better Choices	Poor Choices
Cocktails mixed with club soda, ginger ale, tonic or soft drinks (except colas)	Cocktails mixed with fruit juice, tomato juice, vegetable cocktail, milk, cream or ice cream
Wine, red or white, if potassium is counted (substitute for fruit)	Beer
Non-cola soft drinks such as Sprite, Seven-Up or orange soda	Any cola

Dialysis Diet

Better Choices	**Poor Choices**
Iced tea or coffee	Cocoa, milk, milk shakes, cocoa mixes
Lemonade, limeade, water	Orange juice-type drinks, tomato juice, vegetable juice

Appetizers:
- Look for fresh, simple items to avoid a heavy salt or fluid load before your meal.
- A high-protein appetizer can be used as your main course. Portions are usually smaller and less expensive. Some examples are listed below and will vary with the type of restaurant.

Salads and Salad Bars:
- Salads are often part of the appetizer list. Use your allowed fruits and vegetables for these choices.
- Request that the dressing be served on the side so you can control the amount. Oil and vinegar is always a good choice for dressing. You may bring your own low-

sodium dressing. Lemon or lime juice squeezed generously over the salad can replace salad dressing altogether.
- If they are not listed on the menu, ask the waiter which vegetables or fruits are in the salad. Often these are prepared individually, so you can usually make special requests. Some examples are on page 7.

Better Choices	**Poor Choices**
Caesar salad with chicken or shrimp	Cottage cheese, cheese fondue, other cheese dishes, anchovies
Chicken, pork or steak tostadas	Quiche, cheese sticks
Crab cakes, steamed clams, fried calamari, most shrimp dishes	Oysters
Crab Louis salad	Nachos, potato skins

Dialysis Diet

Better Choices	Poor Choices
Green salad with meat or fish or chef's salad without ham or cheese (request dressing on the side)	Chopped liver or pate; salted or smoked meat, fish or poultry such as ham, lox or smoked turkey soup, bouillion or consomme
Others; meat balls, chicken wings; pot stickers and lumpia (without dipping sauces); fried zucchini, mushrooms or onion rings	

Entrees:

- Portions served in restaurants may be much larger than what you eat at home. When dining out, estimate an amount close to what you normally have. Plan to take the remainder home, or split the meal with another person in your group.

Judy Mitzimberg

Tip: Three ounces of cooked meat, fish or poultry is about the size of a deck of cards. Or, if you weigh meat portions at home, measure them against your hand to use as a guide when eating away from home.

- Grilled items are good choices because you can request how you want them prepared.

Better Choices	Poor Choices
Vegetable salad: lettuce, cabbage, beets, cauliflower, celery, cucumber, jicama, onions, green peas, radishes, sprouts, sweet peppers	Spinach, tomato, avocado, artichoke, kidney beans, garbanzo beans, seeds, nuts
Coleslaw	Potato salad
Beet salad	Three bean salad
Pasta salad, macaroni salad	Greek salad with olives, olive salads, relishes, pickles

Dialysis Diet

Better Choices	Poor Choices
Fruit cup or salad: canned fruit cocktail, canned peaches or pears, fresh or canned pineapple, mandarin oranges	Salad containing melon, oranges, bananas, kiwi, dried fruit
Gelatin salads (plain or with low-potassium fruits or vegetables added)	
Beef (broiled or grilled steaks, burgers without cheese, prime rib roast or hot roast beef sandwiches), chicken (baked, fried, grilled or roasted), leg of lamb, lamb chops, veal, meatloaf	Mixed dishes, beef or lamb stew, liver and onions, cured or salted meats (ham, corned beef, sausage, prossciutto, chorizo)

Better Choices	Poor Choices
Fish or seafood (grilled, steamed or poached)	Bouillabaisse, oysters, lobster newburg, lox
Seafood or meat kabobs	Sauces (especially cheese or tomato), gravies
Fajitas, meat or chicken tacos (no cheese or tomatoes)	Bean dishes, chili beans, chili con carne
Omelets with allowed vegetables and sauce served on the side	Omelets with bacon, cheese, ham, sausage
Sandwiches (request no cheese): roast beef, chicken, egg, turkey, hot roast beef or turkey, fresh seafood sandwich	Submarine sandwich, toasted cheese, BLT, bacon hamburger, Reuben, tuna (canned) salad

- Request that no salt be added when cooking

Dialysis Diet

- Request that gravies or sauces be served on the side
- Avoid mixed dishes or casseroles, which are usually higher in sodium and phosphorus.
- Remove the skin from poultry and any crusts from fried foods to decrease the sodium content.
- It is best NOT to add steak sauce, Worcestershire sauce, soy sauce or hot sauce because of the high sodium content.
- Lemon or lime juice and vinegar are good sauces and will bring out a lot of the true natural flavor of foods. Black pepper will add zest to the food without making you thirsty.

Side Dishes:

The more familiar you are with your diet, the easier it will be to choose appropriate foods. It might be wise to review your food lists before going out.

- Choose starches and vegetables that are lower in potassium such as rice, noodles

and green beans.
- Request a substitute on the menu if necessary.

Better Choices	Poor Choices
Noodles or pasta, pesto pasta, macaroni salad	Spaghetti in tomato sauce
Steamed rice, rice pilaf, rice with peas	Yams, sweet potatoes, fried rice, white potatoes
Unsalted breadsticks, bread or rolls	Baked or barbequed beans, refried beans (refrijoles)
Lower-potassium vegetables like asparagus, cabbage, cooked carrots, corn, eggplant, green peas, zucchini, corn-on-the-cob, coleslaw, lettuce salad	Higher-potassium vegetables like tomatoes, spinach, collard greens, artichokes, acorn squash, etc.

Dialysis Diet

- Ask that sauces be omitted or served on the side

Tip: To increase your choices, avoid higher-potassium fruits and vegetables during the day before eating out.

Better Choices	Poor Choices
Angel food, apple, lemon, pound, spice, white or yellow cake may be topped with whipped cream and low potassium fruit	Cakes rich in chocolate, coconut, dried fruit or nuts, such as carrot, chocolate mousse, devil's food, fruit or German chocolate cake.
Sugar cookies, Lorna Doones, vanilla wafers, lemon creme and butter cookies	Brownies, chocolate, coconut macaroons, snickerdoodles
Fruit ice, sherbet, sorbet	Ice cream or frozen yogurt

Judy Mitzimberg

Better Choices	**Poor Choices**
Lower-potassium fruit desserts like berries, strawberry shortcake, gelatin desserts	Fruits higher in potassium like bananas, oranges or kiwi
Pies, tarts or cobblers made with apple, blueberry, cherry, lemon meringue or strawberry	Pies like banana cream, chocolate cream, coconut, minced meat, pecan, pumpkin, sweet potato or cheesecake

Desserts:
- Ask for a clear description of the dessert. Choose from those desserts that have simple preparations to avoid "hidden" phosphorus and potassium
- Choices with chocolate, cream cheese, ice cream or nuts will be much higher in potassium and phosphorus. Avoid these, share with a friend, or just eat a small amount.

Dialysis Diet

- Remember desserts such as fruit ice, gelatin, sorbet and sherbet add to your fluid intake for the day.
- Sweets may or may not be desirable for you. Always follow the advice of your dietitian who is more familiar with your individual needs.

Remember to take your phosphate binder (also called a phosphorus binder) with your meal. Be sure to carry it with you and keep some in the car so it is always easily available.

Judy Mitzimberg

Specialized or ethnic restaurants

An enjoyable aspect of eating out is trying different ethnic and regional foods. Follow these suggestions for making wise choices.

Chinese Caution: May be very high in sodium

- Request no MSG (monosodium glutamate), soy or fish sauce in food preparation (the menu may include this information.)
- Avoid restaurants that cook in "bulk;" look for those that prepare foods individually. You may call in advance to get this information.
- Avoid adding soy sauce to the food after it is served. Most Chinese restaurants will provide a hot pepper oil. This can be added to make the food spicier, if desired.
- Soups served with the meal are usually high in sodium and may add undesired fluid to weight.
- Choose lower-potassium vegetables such as snow peas, string beans, water

chestnuts, bean sprouts and bok choy. Request stir fried vegetables that are not served in heavy sauces.
- Steamed rice is more authentic and has less sodium than fried rice.
- The tea is often served in a pot on the table. Control the amount poured into your cup to help control your fluid weight gain.
- Enjoy your fortune cookie knowing you have made the best of choices.

French Caution: May be very high in phosphorus

- French restaurants usually use fresh ingredients, but cream and butter may be added in large amounts.
- Try to avoid those foods prepared in cheese or cream sauces. Careful questioning of the waiter can help you make your decision.
- Choose low-potassium fruits and vegetables, and avoid the high-potassium fried potatoes or *pomme frites*.
- French bread is a good choice, low in

sodium, potassium and phosphorus. The butter served is usually "sweet" or unsalted.
- Select a simple, light vinaigrette for salad dressing.
- Desserts are always a highlight. Look for delicious sorbets (count as fluid), cakes, meringues or fruits, such as plums, berries or cherries, that are not in heavy cream sauces or thickly covered with chocolate.

Mexican Caution: May be very high in potassium.

- Put aside the chips and salsa that might be at the table when you first sit down. Save the sodium and potassium for your meal.
- Order a' la carte, or select entrees that are not served with beans and Spanish rice. Some good items are tacos, tostadas and fajitas.
- Beware of the salsas used. Salsa verde is a green sauce but is made of tomatoes. Salsas made of chili peppers without

tomatoes added are the best choices. Remember, guacamole is made from avocados, which are very high in potassium.
- Tortillas are good bread substitutes. Enjoy them.
- For dessert, try the flan as a dairy substitute or any of the fantastic variety of pastries, which are a good choice because they are low in potassium and phosphorus. Pastries are high in saturated fat, however, so make sure to eat them in moderate portions.

Asian Indian Caution: May be very high in phosphorus.

- Indian meals are often vegetarian. While it is best to avoid the bean dishes, there are many other delicious foods to choose from.
- Enjoy experimenting with different flavors. Masala, tandoori and curry preparations are widely available on menus with both

chicken and vegetable entrees.

- Remember to ask which vegetables are included in dishes, and make low-potassium choices. Ask your dietitian for a list of low potassium vegetables and vegetables to limit. (See National Kidney Foundation's fact sheet *Potassium and Renal Diet.*)
- Yogurt is often served as a side dish or part of side dishes, but remember it is a dairy food and high in phosphorus.
- A large selection of Indian breads, such as fried, baked or roasted varieties, are served with most meals, or are available as separate orders.
- Most desserts contain milk or milk powder in the recipe and will be high in phosphorus. Remember to take your phosphate binder.

Italian Caution: May be very high in potassium.

- Beware of the antipasto appetizer that contains salty sausages and pickled or marinated vegetables. These foods could get your meal off to a salty, high-fat start. Also, pass on the minestrone soup, which is high in salt and potassium.

- Request an oil-and-vinegar dressing for the salad.
- Italian bread is a good bread choice. Dipping the bread in olive oil is a healthy alternative to spreading it with butter because olive oil contains heart healthy fats compared to the high animal fats in butter.
- Tomato sauces are poor choices. But pastas are served with may sauces that are not tomato-based. If you do select one with tomato sauce, request that it be served on the side. Limit cheese and white sauces.
- If you choose pizza, look for a light or vegetarian topping, and request that the tomato sauce and cheese be used lightly. It is best to avoid pepperoni or sausage pizzas, which are high in sodium. Other available toppings may include chicken or

fish, both good choices.
- One tablespoon of shredded Parmesan or Romano cheese may be used for flavor. Pepper flakes may be used liberally.
- Italian ices are good dessert choices, but remember to count them as fluid.

Japanese Caution: May be high in sodium.

- Avoid the salty soups, like miso, served at the beginning of the meal.
- Request on MSG (monosodium glutamate) and avoid the soy sauce.
- Sushi can be a good choice as portions are small. Avoid raw fish choices as they may expose you to parasitic infections. Other rolls available include cucumbers and cooked shrimp, crab or eel.
- Try the yakitori, or food grilled on skewers over a charcoal fire. Foods fried in tempura batter are good choices if not dipped in high-sodium sauces.
- Tofu, or soy bean curd, is used regularly in Japanese cooking. It is substituted for

meat in the kidney diet. Be aware that it is often cooked with soy sauce for added flavor.
- The Japanese steak house offers good choices of grilled meat and vegetables, but portions may be large.
- Green tea ice cream is a popular dessert, and is a milk substitute.

Soul Food Caution: May be high in sodium, potassium and phosphorus.

- Soul food is very challenging to the kidney diet because it is frequently high in sodium, potassium and phosphorus as well as fat.
- Salted and cured meats such as ham, sausages, bacon and salt pork should be avoided. Bacon and bacon fat are used extensively in the cooking.
- Organ meats, such as chitterlings, are higher in phosphorus than cuts of muscle meat. Limit these to occasional use.
- Dried beans and black-eyed peas are high

in phosphorus and potassium. Limit these to small amounts (1-2 tablespoons).

- Cooked greens and spinach are popular. Both are high-potassium vegetables. Mustard greens are slightly lower in potassium.
- Yams and sweet potato pie are high in potassium.
- Best choices might include fried chicken (with skin removed), corn, string beans or okra, wilted lettuce, corn bread, butter and sweet potato pie (small wedge). Enjoy, and don't forget your phosphate binders.

Fast Foods

Eating at fast-food restaurants is not totally out of the question. It does, however, take some thought and planning. While many fast-food items are pre-salted, you can ask that yours be prepared without salt. You can also omit the high-sodium condiments such as BBQ or soy sauce and limit others, such as catsup, to one package.

Dialysis Diet

Many fast-food restaurants provide nutrition information so you can check the sodium and potassium content. Your kidney dietitian can also provide this information and tell you the specific amounts of sodium and potassium allowed in your diet.

Better Choices	Poor Choices
Regular or junior size hamburgers	Large, super-or king-size hamburgers or cheeseburgers
Roast beef or turkey sandwiches	Sandwiches with bacon, sauces or cheese
Grilled or broiled chicken sandwiches Tuna or chicken salad	Fried or breaded chicken sandwiches, chicken nuggets or strips
Unsalted onion rings	French fries, tater tots, potato chips, baked potato, potato salad, baked beans

Better Choices	**Poor Choices**
Lettuce salads, coleslaw, macaroni salad	High-potassium foods from the salad bar or pickles; limit tomatoes
Non-cola soda, lemonade, tea and coffee, water	Milk shakes and cola sodas

Dialysis Diet

Emergency Meal Plan
For Times When You Can't Dialyze

What if you can't dialyze due to transportation, power or water problems, bad weather, or some other disaster?

What can you eat and drink to keep your blood values within normal limits until you can dialyze again?

This Emergency Meal Plan will work for short periods of time (five days or less) when you cannot dialyze. This diet is stricter than the diet you usually follow. Remember, you will only be using this diet for a few days until you can dialyze again.

The Emergency Meal Plan is not a Substitute for Dialysis

Choose from these foods only. If a food is not on the list, do not eat it.

Judy Mitzimberg

Guidelines:

1. Limit your meat intake to 3-4 servings each day. The amounts listed below are 1/2 of what you normally eat.

2. Avoid all high potassium fruits and vegetables.

3. Decrease your fluid intake to 1-2 cups each day. Taking in more fluids that this may lead to serious problems.

4. Choose low-salt foods and do not use salt.

5. Use fats and sugars for extra calories, if you need them.

6. If the power is off for a day or more, eat foods in your refrigerator the first day. Eat foods in your freezer while they still have ice crystals in the center. Open your refrigerator or freezer as little as possible, usually only at meal times, to extend the time food will keep.

Dialysis Diet

Each item listed below counts as one choice. The serving sizes may be different from food to food, but each one counts as one serving. Limit yourself to the number of daily servings noted

Meats and Protein Foods:

3-4 choices each day
(about 1/2 of what you would normally eat)

1 egg
1 ounce meat, fish, or poultry
1/4 cup unsalted canned tuna, chicken, or turkey
2 tablespoons unsalted peanut butter
1/4 cup cottage cheese
1 ounce tofu
1/2 can supplement (Boost Plus, Ensure Plus, Nepro)

Dairy Foods:

1 choice each day

1/2 cup sour cream
1 1/2 tablespoons powdered milk
1/2 cup milk

Judy Mitzimberg

Starch:

6 choices each day

1 slice white bread
1/2 English muffin or bagel
5 unsalted crackers
4 slices melba toast
2 graham crackers
6 shortbread cookies or vanilla wafers
1 cup unsalted rice, noodles, or pasta
1 cup puffed wheat, rice, or shredded wheat
1 cup cream of wheat or rice cereal

Vegetables:

1 choice each day
1/2 cup serving

- Green beans
- Zucchini
- Corn
- Beets
- Carrots
- Peas
- Summer squash

Dialysis Diet

Fruits:

4 choices each day
1/2 cup serving

- Plums
- Cherries
- Blackberries
- Raspberries
- Blueberries
- Pineapple
- Strawberries
- Canned pears
- Canned applesauce

Or

- 1 small apple
- 15 grapes

Fats and Oils:

6 or more choices each day
1 teaspoon
- Butter
- Margarine

- Mayonnaise
- Vegetable oil

Fluids:

1 choice
(Plus an amount equal to the total amount of urine produced in a day)

1 cup water, coffee, tea, soda, beer, wine, or milk.

1/2 cup juice (Tang, Kool Aid, High C, cranberry, apple, or grape).

1/2 can supplement (Boost Plus, Ensure Plus, Nepro).

1/2 c. milk or half-and-half.

1/2 cup evaporated milk.

1/2 cup non-dairy creamer, rice or soy milk.

High Calorie Foods:

■	Hard candy	1 piece
■	Jellybeans	10 pieces
■	Marshmallows	1 cup
■	Jam	1 tablespoon
■	Jelly	1 tablespoon

Dialysis Diet

- Honey   1 tablespoon
- Maple syrup   1 tablespoon
- Sugar   1 tablespoon

Special Information for Diabetics:

- Avoid highly-concentrated sweets such as candy; use fats and oils for extra calories.
- Plain cookies, donuts, and cakes are fine when eaten with meals.
- Use unsweetened canned fruit juices, sugar-free Kool-Aid, or diet soda pop.
- Avoid alcohol.
- Have sugar, honey, or juice handy for a low-blood sugar reaction.
- Have several tubes of prepared cake frosting on hand. It can be squeezed into your mouth easily if you have a low-blood sugar reaction.

Emergency Food Supply Ideas:

- Canned unsalted tuna, chicken or turkey.
- Unsalted peanut butter.
- Boost Plus/Ensure Plus/Nepro
- Jam

- Popcorn (unsalted)
- Soy or rice milk
- Bottled water
- Juice mix
- Crackers
- Plain cookies
- Pasta
- Rice
- Cereal
- Canned fruits and vegetables
- Candy (gumdrops, jellybeans)

Emergency Kit:

This emergency kit is designed to help you prepare meals easily in the event that you cannot reach your kitchen.

Have the following items stored in a box that you can reach easily:

- Three days of breakfast, lunch, and dinner menus.
- A can opener.
- 2 plastic gallon jugs of distilled water.

Dialysis Diet

- Bleach - use 1 tablespoon per gallon of water.
- A flashlight and extra batteries.
- A sharp knife.
- Matches in a water-proof container.
- Aluminum foil for storing leftovers.
- Three plastic mixing containers with lids.
- Measuring cups.
- Eating utensils.
- A battery operated transistor radio.
- One week's supply of your personal medications kept in a handy area (this would include such items as blood pressure medicine and phosphate binders). Remember that insulin and some other medications must be kept refrigerated.

Emergency Kit Storage Tips:

- Store the items in a clean, dry place such as in a new garbage can with wheels or in a rubber tub.
- Put labels on the food with dates noting when each item was placed in the emergency kit. Replace items after 1 year.

Judy Mitzimberg

<u>Vascular Access Site Care</u>

Your vascular access (VA) is your lifeline from your vascular system to the dialysis machine. It allows the blood to leave your body, be cleansed and then returned to your body. Having an access that functions well is important to providing adequate dialysis. Without adequate dialysis you will become "uremic". Uremia is the build up of waste products in your blood from the foods you eat.

Whether you have a fistula, graft, or catheter, site care is extremely important. It is your responsibility to care for your vascular access between dialysis treatments.

You can do several things to protect your access:

- Make sure your nurse or technician checks your access before each treatment.

- If you ever notice any redness, swelling, drainage, or heat at the access site, call your surgeon or nephrologist immediately.

- Keep your access clean at all times.

Dialysis Diet

- Use your access site only for dialysis.

- Be careful not to bump or cut your access.

- Don't let anyone put a blood pressure cuff on your access arm.

- Don't wear tight jewelry or tight clothes over your access site.

- Don't sleep with your access arm under your head or body.

- Don't lift heavy objects or put pressure on your access arm.
- Check the pulse in your access every day.

Judy Mitzimberg

Part 2 - Food Values
Introduction

The **Renal Diet** is in a class by itself, as you are well aware if you are on one.

Food values are the break down of the nutritional composition of foods. On the following pages, you will find the protein, sodium, potassium, and phosphorus content of most of the foods you will be eating, measured in grams for protein and milligrams for sodium, potassium, and phosphorus. These charts are designed to assist you in the task of monitoring your intake of these minerals to comply with the guidelines set down by your personal physician.

Have your dietitian fill in the following blanks so when you are planning your meals you will know how much protein, sodium, potassium and phosphorus you are allowed in your daily diet. Knowing your own restrictions will give more meaning to the food value charts.

Dialysis Diet

Daily Allowances:
(To be completed by Renal Dietitian)

- Your daily requirement of calories is: _____calories.

- Your daily requirement of protein is: _____grams.

- Your daily allowance of sodium is: _____milligrams.

- Your daily allowance of potassium is: _____milligrams.

- Your daily allowance of phosphorus is: _____milligrams.

Special dietary instructions:_____
_____
_____
_____
_____
_____
_____

Judy Mitzimberg

Daily Food Guide:
(To be completed by Renal Dietitian)

_____ Ounces of protein per day

_____ Fluid ounces per day

_____ Fat servings per day

_____ Fruit servings per day

_____ Vegetable servings per day

_____ Sweet servings per day

_____ Breads or grains servings Per day

Additional instructions:_____
_____
_____
_____
_____
_____

Dialysis Diet

Following the renal diet prescribed by your doctor and dietitian, going to dialysis and taking your medications will give you the opportunity to be your best every day.

Eating right on dialysis is serious business. If you don't follow your diet you may experience nausea/vomiting, muscle wasting, weakness and fatigue. You may also experience itching, swelling or edema, low blood count, and high blood pressure.

It is extremely important that you have your renal dietitian complete the meal plan on the two previous pages and that you follow it every day. Your dietitian will help you choose the foods that are best for you.

Judy Mitzimberg

Beverages:

	Pro	Na	K	P
Beer, Light - 12 oz	0.71	11	64	42
Beer, regular - 12 oz.	1.07	18	89	43
Club soda - 12 oz.	0.00	75	7	0
Chocolate flavor beverage mix - 2-3 t.	0.71	45	128	28
Chocolate powder prepared w/milk - 1 c.	8.78	165	497	255
Cocoa mix, powder - 1/2 oz. envelope	3.77	168	405	134
Cocoa mix w/aspartame - 1 serving	3.84	173	405	134
Cocoa mix w/o added nutrients - 3 heaping t.	3.06	143	202	89
Cocoa mix w/o nutrients, prepared w/water - 8 oz.	3.09	148	202	89
Coffee, espresso, restaurant prepared - 2 oz.	0.01	8	69	4

Dialysis Diet

Beverages:

	Pro	Na	K	P
Coffee, prepared w/tap water - 6 oz.	0.18	4	96	2
Cola w/caffeine - 12 oz.	0.00	15	4	44
Daiquiri, prepared from recipe - 2 oz.	0.06	3	13	4
Diet cola w/caffeine - 12 oz.	0.36	21	0	32
Diet soda other than cola or pepper type w/caffeine - 12 oz.	0.36	21	7	0
Distilled spirits, all, 80 proof - 1.5 oz.	0.00	0	1	2
Eggnog - 1 c.	9.68	137	419	277
Ginger ale - 12 oz.	0.00	26	4	0
Grape soda - 12 oz.	0.00	56	4	0
Lemonade, frozen concentrate, prepared w/water - 8 oz.	0.25	7	37	5

Judy Mitzimberg

Beverages:

	Pro	**Na**	**K**	**P**
Lemonade flavored drink, powder - 8 oz.	0.00	19	3	3
Lemon-lime soda - 12 oz.	0.00	40	4	0
Malted milk flavored mix, chocolate - 3 t.	1.03	125	251	84
Malted milk flavored mix, natural, prepared w/milk - 1 c.	9.81	204	572	307
Malted milk flavored mix, prepared w/milk - 1 c.	9.01	244	620	313
Malted milk flavored mix, natural powder - 4-5 t.	1.85	85	203	79
Orange soda - 12 oz.	0.00	45	7	4
Pepper type soda w/caffeine - 12 oz.	0.00	37	4	40
Pina colada, prepared from recipe - 4.5 oz.	0.59	8	100	11
Root beer soda - 12 oz.	0.00	48	4	0

Dialysis Diet

Beverages:

	Pro	Na	K	P
Tea, brewed, prepared w/tap water - 6 oz.	0.00	5	66	2
Tea, herb, chamomile, brewed - 6 oz.	0.00	2	16	0
Tea, herb, other than chamomile - 6 oz.	0.00	2	16	0
Tea, instant, lemon flavor w/saccharin - 8 oz.	0.00	24	40	2
Tea, instant, lemon flavor w/sugar - 8 oz.	0.26	8	49	3
Tea, instant, unsweetened - 8 oz.	0.00	7	47	2
Wine, dessert, dry - 3.5 oz.	0.21	9	95	9
Wine, dessert, sweet - 3.5 oz.	0.21	9	95	9
Wine, table, red - 3.5 oz.	0.21	5	115	14
Wine, table, white - 3.5 oz.	0.10	5	82	14

Judy Mitzimberg

Breads:

	Pro	Na	K	P
Biscuits, homemade - 2 1/2"	4.20	348	73	98
Biscuits, homemade - 4"	7.07	586	122	166
Biscuits, refrigerated dough, high fat - 2 1/2"	1.81	325	42	104
Biscuits, refrigerated dough, low-fat - 2 1/4"	1.64	305	39	98
Bread crumbs, dry, grated, plain - 1 oz.	3.54	244	63	42
Bread crumbs, dry, grated, seasoned - 1/4 c.	4.26	795	81	40
Bread stuffing, dry mix, prepared - 1/4 c.	3.20	543	74	42
Bread, banana, homemade - 1 slice	2.58	181	80	35
Bread, cornbread, dry mix, prepared - 1 pc.	4.32	467	77	226
Bread, cornbread, homemade w/2% milk - 1 pc.	4.36	428	96	110

Dialysis Diet

Breads:

	Pro	Na	K	P
Bread, cracked wheat - 1 slice	2.18	135	44	38
Bread, egg - 1/2" slice	3.80	197	46	42
Bread, French, Vienna, sourdough - 1/2" slice	2.20	152	28	26
Bread, Indian fry - (5) 1/2" bread	5.68	556	59	125
Bread, Indian fry - 5" bread	6.39	626	67	141
Bread, Italian - 1 slice	1.76	117	22	21
Bread, mixed grain - 1 slice	2.60	127	53	46
Bread, mixed grain, toasted - 1 slice	2.62	127	53	46
Bread, oatmeal - 1 slice	2.27	162	38	34
Bread, pita, white - 4" pita	2.55	150	34	27

Judy Mitzimberg

Breads:

	Pro	**Na**	**K**	**P**
Bread, pita, white - 6 1/2"	5.46	322	72	58
Bread, pumpernickel - 1 slice	2.78	215	67	57
Bread, pumpernickel, toasted - 1 slice	2.76	214	66	57
Bread, raisin - 1 slice	2.05	101	59	28
Bread, raisin, toasted - 1 slice	2.06	102	59	28
Bread, rye, reduced calorie - 1 slice	2.09	93	23	18
Bread, wheat - 1 slice	2.28	133	50	38
Bread, wheat, reduced calorie - 1 slice	2.09	118	28	23
Bread, white - 1 slice	2.05	135	30	24
Bread, white, toasted - 1 slice	1.98	130	29	23

Dialysis Diet

Breads:

	Pro	Na	K	P
Bread, white, reduced calorie - 1 slice	2.00	104	17	28
Bread, whole wheat - 1 slice	2.72	148	71	64
Bread, whole wheat, toasted - 1 slice	2.73	148	71	65
Crackers, cheese, regular - 10 crackers	1.01	100	15	22
Crackers, cheese w/peanut butter - 1 sandwich	0.88	69	17	23
Crackers, matzo, plain - 1	2.84	1	32	25
Crackers, melba toast, plain - 4 pcs.	2.42	166	40	39
Crackers, rye wafers, plain - 1 wafer	1.06	87	54	37
Crackers, saltines - 4 crackers	1.10	156	15	13
Crackers, standard snack type - 4 crackers	0.85	102	16	27

Judy Mitzimberg

Breads:

	Pro	Na	K	P
Crackers, w/cheese filling - 1 sandwich	0.65	98	30	28
Crackers, wheat, regular - 4 crackers	0.69	64	15	18
Crackers, whole wheat - 4 crackers	1.41	105	48	47
Croissants, butter - 1 croissant	4.67	424	67	60
Croutons, seasoned - 1 c.	4.32	495	72	56
English muffin, plain - 1 muffin	4.39	264	75	76
English muffin, plain, toasted - 1 muffin	4.37	262	74	75
French toast, frozen - 1 slice	4.37	292	79	82
French toast, homemade w/2% milk - 1 slice	5.01	311	87	76
Muffin, blueberry, commercial - 1 muffin	3.14	255	70	112

Dialysis Diet

Breads:

	Pro	Na	K	P
Muffin, blueberry, homemade w/2% milk - 1 muffin	3.71	251	70	83
Muffin, corn, commercial - 1 muffin	3.36	297	39	162
Muffin, corn, dry mix, prepared - 1 muffin	3.70	398	66	192
Muffin, oat bran - 1 muffin	3.99	224	289	214
Muffin, wheat bran w/raisins, toasted - 1 muffin	1.87	179	60	97
Pancakes, plain, frozen - 1 pancake	1.87	183	26	134
Pancakes, dry mix, complete - 1 pancake	1.98	239	67	127
Rolls, hamburger or hotdog - 1 roll	3.66	241	61	38
Rolls, hard (includes kaiser) - 1 roll	5.64	310	62	57
Rolls, dinner, commercial - 1 roll	2.35	146	37	32

Judy Mitzimberg

Breads:

	Pro	Na	K	P
Sweet rolls, homemade, cinnamon w/raisins - 1 roll	3.72	230	67	46
Sweet rolls, cinnamon, refrigerated dough w/frosting - 1 roll	1.62	250	19	104
Taco shells, baked - 1 med.	0.96	49	24	33
Toaster pastry, brown sugar and cinnamon - 1 pastry	2.55	212	57	67
Toaster pastry, fruit - 1 pastry	2.44	218	58	58
Toaster pastry, Kellogg's Pop Tart - 1 pastry	2.65	203	82	44
Tortillas, ready-to-bake or fry, corn - 1 tortilla	1.48	42	40	82
Tortillas, ready-to-bake or fry, flour - 1 tortilla	2.78	153	42	40
Waffle, plain, frozen, toasted - 1 waffle	2.05	260	42	139
Waffle, plain, homemade - 1 waffle	5.93	383	119	143

Dialysis Diet

Candy:

	Pro	Na	K	P
Caramels - 1 pc.	0.46	25	22	12
Caramel/chocolate roll - 1 pc.	0.13	6	7	3
Carob - 1 oz.	2.31	30	179	36
Fudge, homemade - 1 pc.	0.29	11	18	10
Fudge w/nuts, homemade - 1 pc.	0.65	11	30	18
Fudge, vanilla, homemade - 1 pc.	0.18	11	8	5
Fudge, vanilla w/nuts, homemade - 1 pc.	0.44	9	17	11
Gumdrops - 1 med.	0.00	2	0	1
Gumdrops - 10 bears	0.00	10	1	0
Gumdrops - 10 worms	0.00	33	4	0

Judy Mitzimberg

Candy:

	Pro	**Na**	**K**	**P**
Hard candy - 1 pc.	0.00	2	0	0
Hershey, Kit Kat wafer bar - 1 bar	2.98	32	122	100
Hershey, Mr. Goodbar - 1 bar	5.24	73	219	122
Hershey, Reese's Peanut Butter - 1 pkg. of 2	4.64	143	158	91
Hershey, Special Dark - 1 miniature	0.41	1	25	13
Jellybeans - 10 large	0.00	7	10	1
M&M Mars, M&M Peanuts - 10 pcs.	1.89	10	69	46
M&M's plain - 10 pcs.	0.30	4	19	11
Mars Milky Way - 1 bar	2.75	146	147	26
Mars Milky Way - 1 fun size	0.81	43	43	88

Dialysis Diet

Candy:

	Pro	Na	K	P
Marshmallows - 1 c.	0.90	24	3	4
Milk chocolate - 1 bar	3.04	36	169	95
Milk chocolate peanuts - 10 pcs.	5.24	16	201	85
Milk chocolate raisins - 10 pcs.	0.41	4	51	14
Milk chocolate w/almonds - 1 bar	3.69	30	182	108
Nestle Butterfinger - 1 fun size	0.87	14	27	9
Nestle Crunch - 1 bar	2.64	59	151	89
Semi-sweet chocolate - 1 c.	7.06	18	613	222
Snickers - 1 bar	4.56	152	185	127
Starburst Fruit Chews - 1 pc.	0.02	3	0	0

Judy Mitzimberg

Cereals:
General Mills:

	Pro	Na	K	P
Apple Cinnamon Cheerios - 3/4 c.	5.61	9	124	73
Basic 4 - 1 c.	4.18	323	162	232
Berry Berry Kix - 3/4 c.	1.31	185	24	37
Cheerios - 1 c.	3.14	284	89	114
Cinnamon Toast Crunch - 3/4 c.	1.68	210	44	74
Cocoa Puffs - 1 c.	1.14	181	52	43
Corn Chex - 1 c.	2.18	289	32	22
Golden Grahams - 3/4 c.	1.60	275	53	36
Honey Frosted Wheaties - 3/4 c.	1.71	211	56	54

Dialysis Diet

Cereals:

	Pro	**Na**	**K**	**P**
Honey Nut Cheerios - 1 c.	2.78	259	85	103
Honey Nut Chex - 3/4 c.	1.59	224	27	0
Honey Nut Clusters - 1 c.	5.45	239	171	153
Kix - 1 1/3 c.	1.96	263	41	42
Lucky Charms - 1 c.	2.15	2.03	54	76
Raisin Nut Bran - 1 c.	5.16	246	218	163
Reese's Peanut Butter Puffs - 3/4 c.	2.57	177	62	43
Rice Chex - 1 1/4 c.	1.92	291	36	35
Total - 3/4 c.	2.99	199	97	211
Total Corn Flakes - 1 1/3 c.	1.82	203	34	110

Judy Mitzimberg

Cereals:

	Pro	Na	K	P
Total Raisin Bran - 1 c.	4.00	240	287	259
Trix - 1 c.	0.95	197	18	26
Wheat Chex - 1 c.	3.16	269	116	110
Wheaties - 1 c.	3.24	222	104	95

Kelloggs:

	Pro	Na	K	P
All Bran - 1/2 c.	3.66	61	342	294
Apple Jacks - 1 c.	1.44	134	32	30
Cocoa Krispies - 3/4 c.	1.55	210	60	29
Complete Wheat Bran Flakes - 3/4 c.	3.02	226	175	150

Dialysis Diet

Cereals:

	Pro	**Na**	**K**	**P**
Corn Flakes - 1 c.	1.84	298	25	11
Corn Pops - 1 c.	1.15	123	23	7
Crispix - 1 c.	2.15	240	35	27
Froot Loops - 1 c.	1.47	141	32	21
Frosted Flakes - 3/4 c.	1.21	200	20	8
Product 19 - 1 c.	2.67	216	41	33
Raisin Bran - 1 c.	5.61	354	437	214
Rice Krispies - 1 1/4 c.	2.08	354	42	44
Rice Krispies Treats - 3/4 c.	1.11	190	19	20
Smacks - 3/4 c.	1.76	51	42	40

Judy Mitzimberg

Cereals:

	Pro	Na	K	P
Special K - 1 c.	6.36	250	55	51
Shredded Wheat - 2 biscuits	4.78	3	196	168

Quaker:

	Pro	Na	K	P
Cap 'n Crunch - 3/4 c.	1.35	2.08	35	29
Cap 'n Crunch Crunchberries - 3/4 c.	1.26	190	37	30
Cap 'n Crunch Peanut Butter Crunch - 3/4 c.	1.95	2.04	62	52
100% Natural w/oats, honey, and raisins - 1/2 c.	4.84	11	214	150
100% Natural, low-fat, crispy whole grain w/raisins - 1/2 c.	4.15	129	169	119
Oat Cinnamon Life - 1 c.	4.36	220	113	181

Dialysis Diet

Cereals:

	Pro	Na	K	P
Life, plain - 3/4 c.	3.15	174	79	136
Toasted Oatmeal, Honey Nut - 1 c.	4.89	166	185	166
Rice, puffed, fortified - 1 c.	0.88	0	16	14
Wheat, puffed, fortified - 1 c.	1.76	0	42	43

Cooked Cereals:

	Pro	Na	K	P
Bulgar, cooked - 1 c.	561	9	124	73
Bulgar, dry - 1 c.	17.21	24	574	420
Corn grits, yellow, cooked w/o salt - 1 c.	3.39	0	53	29
Corn grits, white, cooked w/o salt - 1 c.	3.39	0	53	29

Judy Mitzimberg

Cooked Cereals:

	Pro	**Na**	**K**	**P**
Cream of Wheat, mix-n-eat - 1 packet	2.70	241	38	20
Cream of Wheat, quick cooked - 1 c.	3.59	139	45	100
Cream of Wheat, regular, cooked w/o salt - 1 c.	3.77	3	43	43
Malt-O-Meal, cooked w/o salt - 1 c.	3.60	2	31	24
Oat Bran, cooked - 1 c.	7.03	2	201	261
Oat Bran, raw - 1 c.	16.26	4	532	690
Oats, instant, prepared w/water - 1 packet	4.43	285	99	133
Oats, regular, quick and instant - 1 c.	6.08	2	131	178
Quaker corn grits - 1 packet	2.21	289	38	29
Quaker oatmeal, instant, maple and brown surgar - 1 packet	4.17	234	112	132

Dialysis Diet

Cooked Cereals:

	Pro	**Na**	**K**	**P**
Quaker oatmeal, instant, apple and cinnamon - 1 packet	3.19	121	106	113
Wheatena, cooked w/water - 1 c.	4.86	5	187	146

Cheese and Dairy:

	Pro	**Na**	**K**	**P**
Butter w/salt - 1 T.	0.12	117	4	3
Butter w/o salt - 1 T.	0.12	2	4	3
Cheese food, process American - 1 oz.	5.56	337	79	130
Cheese sauce, homemade - 1/2 c.	12.55	599	173	278
Cheese spread, process American - 1 oz.	4.65	381	69	202
Cheese, blue - 1 oz.	6.07	395	73	110

Judy Mitzimberg

Cheese and Dairy:

	Pro	Na	K	P
Cheese, camembert - 1 oz.	7.52	320	71	1321
Cheese, cheddar - 1 oz.	7.06	176	28	145
Cheese, cottage, creamed - 1 c.	26.23	851	176	277
Cheese, cottage, creamed w/fruit - 1 c.	22.37	915	151	237
Cheese, cottage, low-fat 1% milk fat - 1 c.	28.00	918	194	303
Cheese, cottage, low-fat 2% milk fat - 1 c.	31.05	918	217	341
Cheese, cottage, non-fat - 1 c.	25.04	19	46	151
Cheese, cream - 1 T.	1.09	43	17	15
Cheese, cream, fat-free - 1 T.	2.25	85	25	68
Cheese, feta - 1 oz.	4.03	316	18	96

Dialysis Diet

Cheese and Dairy:

	Pro	Na	K	P
Cheese, low-fat cheddar or colby - 1 oz.	6.90	174	19	137
Cheese, mozzarella, part skim milk - 1 oz.	7.79	150	27	149
Cheese, mozzarella, whole milk - 1 oz.	5.51	106	19	105
Cheese, muenster - 1 oz.	6.64	178	38	133
Cheese, neufchatel - 1 oz.	2.82	113	32	39
Cheese, parmesan, grated - 1 T.	2.08	93	5	40
Cheese, pasteurized, process American - 1 oz.	6.28	405	46	211
Cheese, pasteurized, Swiss - 1 oz.	7.01	388	61	216
Cheese, provolone - 1 oz.	7.25	248	39	141
Cheese, ricotta, part skim milk - 1 c.	28.02	308	308	450

Judy Mitzimberg

Cheese and Dairy:

	Pro	**Na**	**K**	**P**
Cheese, ricotta, whole milk - 1 c.	27.70	207	258	389
Cheese, Swiss - 1 oz.	8.06	74	31	172
Cheesecake, commercial - 1 slice	4.40	166	72	74
Cream, fluid, half and half - 1 T.	0.44	6	20	14
Cream, fluid, heavy whipping - 1 T.	0.31	6	11	9
Cream, fluid, light (coffee cream) - 1 T.	0.41	6	18	12
Cream, fluid, light whipping - 1 T.	0.33	5	15	9
Cream, sour, cultured - 1 T.	0.38	6	17	10
Cream, sour, reduced fat, cultured - 1 T.	0.44	6	19	14
Cream, whipped, pressurized - 1 T.	0.10	4	4	3

Dialysis Diet

Cheese and Dairy:

	Pro	Na	K	P
Dessert topping, powdered, prepared w/1/2 c. milk - 1 T.	0.14	3	6	3
Dessert topping, pressurized - 1 T.	0.04	2	1	1
Dessert topping, semi-solid, frozen - 1 T.	0.05	1	1	0
Margarine, regular w/salt - 1 T.	0.13	133	6	3
Margarine, soft w/salt - 1 t.	0.04	51	2	1
Margarine-butter blend, 60% corn oil margarine, 40% butter - 1 T.	0.12	127	5	3
Margarine-like spread, 40% fat - 1 t.	0.02	46	1	1
Margarine-like spread, 60% fat, stick - 1 t.	0.03	48	1	2
Margarine-like spread, 60% fat, stick - 1 T.	0.09	143	4	1

Judy Mitzimberg

Cheese and Dairy:

	Pro	Na	K	P
Milkshake, thick, chocolate - 10.6 oz.	9.15	333	672	378
Milkshake, thick, vanilla - 11 oz.	12.08	297	573	360
Milk, buttermilk, dried - 1 T.	2.23	34	103	61
Milk, buttermilk, fluid, cultured, low-fat - 1 c.	8.11	257	370	218
Milk, canned, sweetened - 1 c.	24.20	389	1135	774
Milk, evaporated, non-fat - 1 c.	19.33	294	850	499
Milk, evaporated w/o vitamin A - 1 c.	17.16	267	764	512
Milk, chocolate, commercial - 1 c.	7.93	150	418	253
Milk, chocolate, commercial, low-fat - 1 c.	8.10	153	425	258
Milk, chocolate, commercial, reduced fat - 1 c.	8.03	150	423	255

Dialysis Diet

Cheese and Dairy:

	Pro	Na	K	P
Milk, dry, non-fat w/vitamin A - 1/3 c.	8.07	126	392	227
Milk, fluid, 3/25 milk fat - 1 c.	8.03	120	371	227
Milk, fluid, low-fat, 1% w/vitamin A - 1 c.	8.03	124	381	234
Milk, fluid, non-fat (fat free, skim) - 1 c.	8.35	127	407	247
Milk, fluid, reduced fat, 2% - 1 c.	8.13	122	376	232
Yogurt, fruit, low-fat - 8 oz.	9.92	132	443	270
Yogurt, plain, low-fat - 8 oz.	11.92	159	531	327
Yogurt, plain, skim milk - 8 oz.	13.01	175	579	356
Yogurt, plain, whole milk - 8 oz.	7.88	104	352	216

Desserts:

Cake:

	Pro	Na	K	P
Angelfood cake, commercial - 1 pc.	1.65	210	26	9
Angelfood cake, dry mix, prepared - 1 pc.	3.05	255	68	116
Boston cream pie, commercial - 1 pc.	2.21	132	36	45
Chocolate cake w/frosting, commercial - 1 pc.	2.62	214	128	78
Chocolate cake, homemade w/o frosting - 1 pc.	5.04	299	133	101
Coffeecake, cinnamon, commercial - 1 pc.	4.28	221	77	68
Fruitcake, commercial - 1 pc.	1.25	116	66	22
Gingerbread, homemade - 1 pc.	2.89	242	325	40
Pineapple upside down cake, homemade - 1 pc.	4.03	367	129	94

Dialysis Diet

Desserts:

	Pro	Na	K	P
Pound cake, commercial - 1 pc.	1.54	111	33	38
Pound cake, fat-free - 1 pc.	1.51	95	31	41
Shortcake, biscuit type - 1 biscuit	3.97	329	69	93
Snack cake, cream filled w/frosting - 1 cake	1.70	213	61	47
Snack cake, cream filled, sponge - 1 cake	1.32	155	37	79
Snack cake w/frosting, low-fat - 1 cake	1.85	178	96	79
Sponge cake, commercial - 1 pc.	1.62	73	30	41
Sponge cake, homemade - 1 pc.	4.60	144	89	63
White cake, homemade, w/frosting - 1 pc.	4.93	318	111	78
Yellow cake, commercial, w/frosting - 1 pc.	2.43	216	114	103

Judy Mitzimberg

Desserts:
Cookies:

	Pro	**Na**	**K**	**P**
Brownies, commercial - 1	2.69	175	83	57
Brownies, dry mix, prepared - 1	0.84	21	69	11
Butter cookies, commercial - 1	0.31	18	6	5
Chocolate chip, commercial - 1	0.54	32	14	11
Chocolate chip, low-fat, commercial - 1	0.58	38	12	8
Chocolate chip, homemade w/margarine - 1	0.91	58	36	16
Chocolate chip, refrigerated dough, baked - 1	1.27	60	52	20
Chocolate sandwich w/cream filling - 1	0.47	60	18	10
Fig bar - 1	0.59	56	33	10

Dialysis Diet

Cookies:

	Pro	Na	K	P
Graham crackers, plain or honey - 2 squares	0.97	85	19	15
Molasses - 1 med.	0.84	69	52	14
Molasses - 1 lg.	1.79	147	111	30
Oatmeal, fat-free, commercial - 1	0.65	33	23	12
Oatmeal, regular, commercial - 1	1.55	96	36	35
Oatmeal, homemade w/raisins - 1	0.98	81	36	24
Oatmeal, soft type, commercial - 1	0.92	52	20	31
Peanut butter, commercial - 1	1.44	62	25	13
Peanut butter, homemade - 1	1.80	104	46	23
Shortbread pecan, commercial - 1	0.69	39	10	12

Judy Mitzimberg

Cookies:

	Pro	Na	K	P
Shortbread, plain, commercial - 1	0.49	36	8	9
Sugar, commercial - 1	0.77	54	9	12
Sugar, homemade w/margarine - 1	0.83	69	11	13
Sugar, refrigerated dough, baked - 1	0.71	70	24	28
Vanilla sandwich w/cream filling - 1	0.68	52	14	11
Vanilla wafers, lower-fat - 1	0.20	12	4	4

Dialysis Diet

Miscellaneous Desserts:

	Pro	Na	K	P
Danish pastry, cheese - 1	5.68	320	70	77
Danish pastry, fruit - 1	3.83	251	59	63
Chocolate pudding, dry mix, instant prepared w/2% milk - 1/2 c.	4.56	417	1	30
Chocolate pudding, regular, w/2% milk - 1/2 c.	4.69	149	0	32
Chocolate pudding, ready-to-eat - 4 oz.	3.05	146	247	353
Rice pudding, ready-to-eat - 4 oz.	2.27	96	240	138
Tapioca pudding, ready-to-eat - 4 oz.	2.26	180	203	90
Vanilla pudding, dry, regular, prepared w/2% milk - 1/2 c.	4.20	224	68	77
Vanilla pudding, ready-to-eat - 4 oz.	2.60	153	110	89

Judy Mitzimberg

Miscellaneous Desserts:

	Pro	Na	K	P
Doughnuts, cake type, plain - 1 hole	0.70	76	18	38
Doughnuts, cake type, plain - 1 med.	2.35	257	60	126
Doughnuts, yeast, glazed - 1 hole	0.83	44	14	12
Doughnuts, yeast, glazed - 1 med.	3.84	205	65	56
Eclairs, custard filled - 1	6.40	337	117	107
Frozen fruit and juice bars - 1 bar	0.92	3	41	5
Ice cream, chocolate - 1/2 c.	2.51	50	164	71
Ice cream, French vanilla - 1/2 c.	3.53	52	152	100
Ice cream, light, 50% less fat, vanilla - 1/2 c.	2.51	56	139	72
Ice cream, vanilla - 1/2 c.	2.31	53	131	69

Dialysis Diet

Miscellaneous Desserts:

	Pro	Na	K	P
Ice Pops - 1 bar	0.00	7	2	0
Ice, Italian, restaurant prepared - 1/2 c.	0.03	5	7	0
Sherbet, orange - 1/2 c.	0.81	34	71	30
Frozen yogurt, chocolate, soft serve - 1/2 c.	2.88	71	188	100
Frozen yogurt, vanilla, soft serve - 1/2 c.	2.88	63	152	93

Pies:

	Pro	Na	K	P
Apple, commercial - 1 pc.	2.22	311	76	28
Apple, homemade - 1 pc.	3.72	327	122	43
Blueberry, commercial - 1 pc.	2.11	380	59	27

Judy Mitzimberg

Pies:

	Pro	**Na**	**K**	**P**
Blueberry, homemade - 1 pc.	3.97	272	74	44
Cherry, commercial - 1 pc.	2.34	288	95	34
Cherry, homemade - 1 pc.	5.04	344	139	54
Chocolate cream, commercial - 1 pc.	2.94	154	144	77
Coconut custard, commercial - 1 pc.	6.14	348	182	127
Fried pies, fruit - 1 pie	3.84	479	83	55
Lemon meringue, commercial - 1 pc.	1.70	165	101	119
Lemon meringue, homemade - 1 pc.	4.83	307	83	53
Pecan, homemade - 1 pc.	5.98	320	162	115
Pumpkin, homemade - 1 pc.	6.98	349	288	152

Dialysis Diet

Eggs:

	Pro	Na	K	P
Egg substitute, liquid - 1/4 c.	7.53	111	207	76
Egg white, raw, fresh - 1 lg.	3.51	55	48	4
Egg yolk, raw, fresh - 1 lg.	2.78	7	16	81
Egg, whole, raw, fresh - 1 lg.	6.25	63	61	103
Egg, whole, fried - 1 lg.	6.23	162	61	89
Egg, whole, hard boiled - 1 lg.	6.29	62	63	86
Egg, whole, poached - 1 lg.	6.22	140	60	89
Egg, whole, scrambled - 1 lg.	6.76	171	84	104
Eggnog - 1 c.	9.68	137	419	277

Judy Mitzimberg

Entrees - Frozen or Homemade:

	Pro	**Na**	**K**	**P**
Beef stew, homemade - 1 c.	22.00	461	527	233
Chicken and noodles, homemade - 1 c.	22.03	600	149	247
Chicken pot pie, frozen - 1 sm.	13.04	857	256	119
Chile con carne w/beans, canned - 1/2 c.	10.09	516	304	97
Fish fillet, breaded and fried - 1 fillet	13.34	484	291	156
Green pepper, stuffed, homemade - 1 med.	24.01	581	477	224
Oyster stew, homemade - 1 c.	12.05	812	319	266
Pasta w/meatballs in tomato sauce - 1 c.	10.89	1053	416	116
Pizza w/cheese - 1 slice	7.68	336	110	113
Pizza w/cheese, meat and vegetables - 1 slice	13.01	382	179	131

Dialysis Diet

Entrees – Frozen or Homemade:

	Pro	Na	K	P
Pizza w/pepperoni - 1 slice	10.12	267	153	75
Spanish rice, homemade - 1 c.	4.44	774	566	96
Spinach souffle, homemade - 1 c.	10.99	763	201	231
Tostada w/guacamole - 1	6.24	399	325	116

Fast Foods:

	Pro	Na	K	P
Biscuit w/egg and sausage - 1	19.15	1141	320	490
French toast w/butter - 2 slices	10.34	513	177	146
Burrito w/beans and cheese - 1	7.53	593	248	90
Burrito w/beans and meat - 1	11.24	668	328	90

Fast Foods:

	Pro	Na	K	P
Cheeseburger, single, w/condiments and vegetables - 1	15.96	616	223	176
Cheeseburger, double, w/condiments and vegetables - 1	21.25	1051	335	242
Cheeseburger, double, plain - 1	22.13	891	285	338
Chicken fillet sandwich, plain - 1	24.12	957	353	233
Chicken, boneless, breaded and fried - 6 pcs.	18.02	513	305	289
Chili con carne - 1 c.	24.62	1007	691	197
Chimichanga w/beef - 1	19.61	910	586	124
Clams, breaded and fried - 3/4 c.	12.82	834	266	238
Coleslaw - 3/4 c.	1.46	267	177	36
Croissant w/egg, cheese, and bacon - 1	16.23	889	201	276

Dialysis Diet

Fast Foods:

	Pro	Na	K	P
Danish pastry, cheese - 1	5.83	319	116	80
Danish pastry, fruit - 1	4.76	333	110	69
Enchilada w/cheese - 1	9.63	784	240	134
English muffin w/egg, cheese, and Canadian bacon - 1	16.69	729	199	270
Fish sandwich w/tarter and cheese - 1	20.61	939	353	311
French toast sticks - 5 sticks	8.28	499	127	123
Frijoles w/cheese - 1 c.	11.37	882	605	175
Hamburger, lg., double, w/condiments and vegetables - 1	34.28	791	570	314
Hamburger, regular, double w/condiments - 1	31.82	742	527	284
Hamburger, regular, single w/condiments - 1	12.32	534	251	114

Judy Mitzimberg

Fast Foods:

	Pro	Na	K	P
Hot dog, plain - 1	10.39	670	143	97
Hot dog w/chili - 1	13.51	480	166	192
Hot dog w/corn flour coating - 1	16.80	973	263	166
Hush puppies - 5 pcs.	4.88	965	188	190
Ice milk, vanilla w/cone - 1	3.89	92	169	139
Nachos w/cheese - 6-8	9.10	816	172	276
Onion rings, breaded and fried - 8-9	3.70	430	129	86
Pancakes w/butter and syrup - 2	8.26	1104	251	476
Potato, French fried in vegetable oil - 1 sm.	3.66	168	586	110
Potato, French fried in vegetable oil - 1 lg.	7.27	335	1164	173

Dialysis Diet

Fast Foods:

	Pro	Na	K	P
Potato, mashed - 1/3 c.	1.85	182	235	44
Potato, hash browns - 1/2 c.	1.94	290	267	69
Roast beef sandwich, plain - 1	21.50	792	316	239
Salad, vegetable w/cheese and egg w/o dressing - 1 1/2 c.	8.77	119	371	132
Salad, vegetable w/chicken, w/o dressing - 1 1/2 c.	17.44	209	447	170
Shrimp, breaded and fried - 6-8	18.88	1446	184	344
Submarine sandwich w/cold cuts - 6"	21.84	1651	394	287
Submarine sandwich, roast beef - 6"	28.64	845	330	192
Submarine sandwich, tuna salad - 6"	29.70	1293	335	220

Judy Mitzimberg

Fast Foods:

	Pro	**Na**	**K**	**P**
Sundae, hot fudge - 1	5.64	182	395	228
Taco salad - 1 1/2 c.	13.23	762	416	143
Taco, beef - 1 lg.	31.77	1233	729	313
Taco, beef - 1 sm.	20.66	802	474	203
Tostada w/beans, beef and cheese - 1	16.09	871	491	173

Fish:

Catfish, channel, breaded and fried - 3 oz.	15.38	238	289	184
Clams, mixed species, canned - 3 oz.	21.72	95	534	287
Clams, mixed species, raw - 3 oz.	10.85	48	267	144

Dialysis Diet

Fish:

	Pro	Na	K	P
Cod, Atlantic, canned - 3 oz.	19.35	185	449	221
Cod, Pacific, cooked dry heat - 3 oz.	19.51	77	439	190
Crab, Alaska king, cooked moist heat - 3 oz.	16.45	911	223	238
Crab, blue, canned - 1 c.	27.70	450	505	351
Crab, blue, cooked moist heat - 3 oz.	17.17	237	275	175
Crab, blue, crab cakes - 1 cake	12.13	198	194	128
Crab, imitation, made from surimi - 3 oz.	10.22	715	240	77
Fish portions and sticks, frozen, pre-heated - 1 pc.	4.38	163	73	103
Flounder or sole, cooked dry heat - 3 oz.	20.54	89	292	367
Flounder or sole, cooked dry heat - 1 fillet	30.68	133	437	246

Fish:

	Pro	Na	K	P
Haddock, cooked dry heat - 1 fillet	36.36	131	599	362
Haddock, cooked dry heat - 3 oz.	20.60	74	339	205
Halibut, Atlantic or Pacific, cooked dry heat - 3 oz.	22.69	59	490	242
Halibut, cooked dry heat - 1/2 fillet	42.44	110	916	453
Herring, Atlantic, pickled - 3 oz.	12.07	740	59	76
Lobster, Northern, cooked moist heat - 3 oz.	17.43	323	299	157
Ocean perch, Atlantic, cooked dry heat - 3 oz.	20.30	82	298	235
Oysters, Eastern, breaded and fried - 3 oz.	7.45	354	207	135
Oysters, Eastern, wild, raw - 6 med.	5.92	177	131	113
Pollock, walleye, cooked dry heat - 3 oz.	19.98	99	329	289

Dialysis Diet

Fish:

	Pro	**Na**	**K**	**P**
Pollock, walleye, cooked dry heat - 1 fillet	14.11	70	232	410
Rockfish, Pacific, cooked dry heat - 1 fillet	35.82	115	775	194
Rockfish, Pacific, cooked dry heat - 3 oz.	20.43	65	442	340
Roughy, orange, cooked dry heat - 3 oz.	16.02	69	327	218
Salmon, Chinook, smoked - 3 oz.	15.55	667	149	139
Salmon, pink, canned - 3 oz.	16.81	471	277	280
Salmon, sockeye, cooked dry heat - 3 oz.	23.21	56	319	428
Salmon, sockeye, cooked dry heat - 1/2 fillet	42.33	102	581	235
Sardines, Atlantic, canned in oil - 3 oz.	20.94	430	338	417
Scallops, mixed species, breaded and fried - 6 pcs.	16.81	432	310	219

Judy Mitzimberg

Fish:

	Pro	Na	K	P
Swordfish, cooked dry heat - 3 oz.	21.58	98	314	357
Swordfish, cooked dry heat - 1 pc.	26.91	122	391	286
Trout, rainbow, cooked dry heat - 3 oz.	20.63	36	375	226
Tuna salad - 1 c.	32.88	824	365	365
Tuna, light, canned in oil - 3 oz.	24.78	301	176	265
Tuna, light, canned in water - 3 oz.	21.68	287	201	139
Tuna, white, canned in water - 3 oz.	20.08	320	201	184
Tuna, yellow fin, fresh, cooked dry heat - 3 oz.	25.47	40	484	208

Note: A one-minute rinse of 6 1/2 oz. of water-packed canned fish will wash away about 3/4 of the sodium

Dialysis Diet

Fruits:

	Pro	Na	K	P
Apples, dried, sulfured, uncooked - 5 rings	0.30	28	144	12
Apples, raw w/skin - 1	0.26	0	159	10
Apples, raw w/o skin - 1 c.	0.17	0	124	8
Applesauce, canned, sweetened w/o salt - 1 c.	0.46	8	156	18
Applesauce, unsweetened - 1 c.	0.41	5	183	17
Apricots, canned in heavy syrup - 1 c.	1.37	10	361	31
Apricots, canned in juice pack - 1 c.	1.54	10	403	49
Apricots, dried, sulfured, uncooked - 10 halves	1.28	4	482	41
Apricots, raw - 1	0.49	0	104	7
Avacado, raw, California - 1 oz.	0.60	3	180	12

Judy Mitzimberg

Fruits:

	Pro	Na	K	P
Avacado, raw, Florida - 1 oz.	0.45	1	138	11
Banana, raw - 1	1.22	1	467	24
Banana, raw - 1 c.	1.55	2	594	30
Blackberries, raw - 1 c.	1.04	0	282	30
Blueberries, frozen, sweetened - 1 c.	0.92	2	138	16
Blueberries, raw - 1 c.	0.97	9	129	15
Carambola (star fruit), raw - 1 fruit	0.49	2	148	15
Carambola (star fruit), raw - 1 c.	0.58	2	176	17
Cherries, sour, red, water pack - 1 c.	1.88	17	239	24
Cherries, sweet, raw - 10	0.82	0	152	13

Dialysis Diet

Fruits:

	Pro	Na	K	P
Cranberry sauce, canned, sweetened - 1 slice	0.11	17	15	3
Dates, domestic, natural and dry - 5	0.82	1	271	17
Dates, domestic, natural and dry - 1 c.	3.51	5	1161	71
Figs, dried, uncooked - 2	1.16	4	271	26
Fruit butters, apple - 1 T.	0.07	1	15	2
Fruit cocktail, heavy syrup - 1 c.	0.97	15	218	27
Fruit cocktail, juice pack - 1 c.	1.09	9	225	33
Fruit, mixed, frozen, sweetened - 1 c.	3.55	8	328	30
Grapefruit, raw, pink and red - 1/2 grapefruit	0.68	0	159	11
Grapefruit, raw, white - 1/2 grapefruit	0.81	0	175	9

Judy Mitzimberg

Fruits:

	Pro	**Na**	**K**	**P**
Grapefruit sections, canned, light syrup - 1 c.	1.42	5	328	25
Grapes, red and green, raw - 1 c.	1.06	3	296	21
Grapes, red and green, raw - 10	0.33	1	93	7
Kiwi fruit, fresh, raw - 1 med.	0.75	4	252	30
Lemon, raw w/o peel - 1	0.64	1	80	9
Mango, raw - 1	1.06	4	323	23
Mango, raw - 1 c.	0.84	3	257	18
Melon, cantaloupe, raw - 1 c.	1.41	14	494	27
Melon, cantaloupe, raw - 1/8 melon	0.61	6	213	12
Melon, honeydew, raw - 1 c.	0.78	17	461	17

Dialysis Diet

Fruits:

	Pro	Na	K	P
Melon, honeydew, raw - 1/8 melon	0.74	16	434	16
Nectarine, raw - 1	1.28	0	288	22
Oranges, raw, all varieties - 1	1.23	0	237	18
Oranges, raw, all varieties - 1 c.	1.69	0	326	25
Papaya, raw - 1 c.	0.85	4	360	7
Papaya, raw - 1 papaya	1.85	9	781	15
Peaches, canned, heavy syrup - 1 c.	1.18	16	241	29
Peaches, canned, heavy syrup - 1/2 peach	0.44	6	90	11
Peaches, canned, juice pack - 1 c.	1.56	10	317	42
Peaches, canned, juice pack - 1/2 peach	0.62	4	125	17

Judy Mitzimberg

Fruits:

	Pro	Na	K	P
Peaches, dried, uncooked - 3 halves	1.41	3	388	46
Peaches, frozen, sliced, sweetened - 1 c.	1.58	15	325	28
Peaches, raw - 1	0.69	0	193	12
Peaches, raw - 1 c.	1.19	0	335	20
Pears, Asian, raw - 1	1.38	0	333	30
Pears, canned, heavy syrup - 1/2 pear	0.15	4	49	5
Pears, canned, heavy syrup - 1 c.	0.53	13	173	19
Pears, canned, juice pack - 1 c.	0.84	10	238	30
Pears, canned, juice pack - 1/2 pear	0.26	3	73	9
Pears, raw - 1	0.65	0	208	18

Dialysis Diet

Fruits:

	Pro	**Na**	**K**	**P**
Pineapple, canned, heavy syrup - 1 c.	0.89	3	264	18
Pineapple, canned, heavy syrup - 1 slice	0.17	0	51	3
Pineapple, canned, juice pack - 1 slice	0.20	0	57	3
Pineapple, canned, juice pack - 1 c.	1.05	2	304	15
Pineapple, raw - 1 c.	0.60	2	175	11
Plums, purple, heavy syrup - 1	0.17	9	42	6
Plums, purple, heavy syrup - 1 c.	0.93	49	235	34
Plums, purple, juice pack - 1	0.23	0	71	7
Plums, purple, juice pack - 1 c.	1.29	3	388	38
Plums, raw - 1	0.52	0	114	7

Judy Mitzimberg

Fruits:

	Pro	**Na**	**K**	**P**
Prunes, dried, stewed w/o sugar - 1 c.	2.90	5	828	87
Prunes, dried, uncooked - 5 prunes	1.10	2	313	33
Raisins, seedless - 1 c.	4.67	17	1089	141
Raisins, seedless - 1 packet	0.45	2	105	14
Raspberries, frozen, sweetened - 1 c.	1.75	3	285	43
Raspberries, raw - 1 c.	1.12	0	187	15
Rhubarb, frozen, cooked w/sugar - 1 c.	0.94	2	230	19
Strawberries, frozen, sweetened - 1 c.	1.35	8	250	33
Strawberries, raw - 1 berry	0.07	0	20	2
Strawberries, raw - 1 c.	1.01	2	276	32

Dialysis Diet

Fruits:

	Pro	Na	K	P
Tangerines, raw - 1	0.53	1	132	8
Watermelon, raw - 1 wedge	1.77	6	332	26
Watermelon, raw - 1 c.	0.94	3	176	14

Juices:

Apple juice, unsweetened - 1 c.	0.15	7	295	17
Apricot nectar w/ascorbic acid - 1 c.	0.93	8	286	23
Carrot juice, canned - 1 c.	2.24	68	689	99
Cranberry juice cocktail, bottled - 8 oz.	0.00	5	46	5
Fruit punch drink, canned - 8 oz.	0.00	55	62	2

Juices:

	Pro	Na	K	P
Grape drink, canned - 8 oz.	0.00	15	13	3
Grape juice, frozen concentrate, sweetened, diluted w/3 cans water - 1 c.	0.48	5	53	10
Grapefruit juice, canned, sweetened - 1 c.	1.45	5	405	28
Grapefruit juice, canned, unsweetened - 1 c.	1.28	2	378	27
Grapefruit juice, frozen concentrate, unsweetened, diluted w/3 cans water - 1 c.	1.36	2	336	35
Grapefruit juice, pink, raw - 1 c.	1.24	2	400	37
Grapefruit juice, white, raw - 1 c.	1.24	2	400	37
Lemon juice, canned or bottled - 1 T.	0.06	3	16	1

Dialysis Diet

Juices:

	Pro	Na	K	P
Lemon juice, raw - juice of 1 lemon	0.18	0	58	3
Lime juice, canned or bottled, unsweetened - 1 T.	0.04	2	12	2
Lime juice, raw - juice of 1 lime	0.17	0	41	3
Orange juice, canned, sweetened - 1 c.	1.47	5	436	35
Orange juice, frozen concentrate, unsweetened, diluted w/3 cans water - 1 c.	1.69	2	473	40
Orange juice, raw - juice from 1 orange	0.60	1	172	15
Orange juice, raw - 1 c.	1.74	2	496	42
Pineapple grapefruit juice drink - 8 oz.	0.50	35	153	15
Pineapple orange juice drink - 8 oz.	3.25	8	115	10

Judy Mitzimberg

Juices:

	Pro	**Na**	**K**	**P**
Pineapple juice, unsweetened - 1 c.	0.80	3	335	20
Prune juice, canned - 1 c.	1.56	10	707	64
Tomato juice, canned w/salt added - 1 c.	1.85	877	535	46
Vegetable juice cocktail, canned - 1 c.	1.52	653	467	41

Meats:

	Pro	**Na**	**K**	**P**
Beef, chuck blade roast, lean and fat, cooked - 3 oz.	22.58	54	196	170
Beef, chuck blade roast, lean only, cooked - 3 oz.	26.40	60	224	200
Beef, corned beef, canned - 3 oz.	23.05	856	116	94
Beef, cured, dried beef - 1 oz.	8.25	984	126	49

Dialysis Diet

Meats:

	Pro	Na	K	P
Beef, ground, extra lean, cooked - 3 oz.	21.59	60	266	137
Beef, ground, lean, cooked - 3 oz.	21.01	65	256	134
Beef, ground, regular, cooked - 3 oz.	20.46	71	248	145
Beef, rib, whole (6-12 ribs), lean and fat, roasted - 3 oz.	19.13	54	256	149
Beef, rib, whole (6-12 ribs), lean only, roasted - 3 oz.	23.16	61	318	182
Beef, round, bottom round, lean and fat, cooked - 3 oz.	24.36	43	240	208
Beef, round, bottom round, lean only, cooked - 3 oz.	26.85	43	262	231
Beef, round, eye of round, lean and fat, cooked - 3 oz.	22.77	50	308	177
Beef, round, eye of round, lean only, cooked - 3 oz.	24.64	53	366	192
Beef, top sirloin, lean and fat, cooked - 3 oz.	23.64	54	311	189

Judy Mitzimberg

Meats:

	Pro	**Na**	**K**	**P**
Beef, top sirloin, lean only, cooked - 3 oz.	25.81	56	343	207
Beef, liver, pan fried - 3 oz.	22.71	90	309	392
Bologna, beef and pork - 2 slices	6.63	578	102	52
Braunschweiger (a liver sausage) - 2 slices	7.65	648	113	95
Frankfurter, beef - 1 frank	5.40	462	75	39
Frankfurter, beef and pork - 1 frank	5.08	504	75	39
Frankfurter, chicken - 1 frank	5.82	617	38	48
Ham, chopped, not canned - 2 slices	3.60	288	67	33
Ham, sliced, extra lean - 2 slices	10.97	810	198	124
Ham, sliced, regular - 2 slices	9.96	747	188	140

Dialysis Diet

Meats:

	Pro	Na	K	P
Lamb, domestic, leg, lean and fat, roasted - 3 oz.	21.72	56	266	162
Lamb, domestic, leg, lean only, roasted - 3 oz.	24.06	58	287	175
Lamb, domestic, loin, lean and fat, broiled - 3 oz.	21.39	65	278	167
Lamb, domestic, loin, lean only, broiled - 3 oz.	25.49	71	320	192
Lamb, domestic, rib, lean and fat, roasted - 3 oz.	17.95	62	230	141
Lamb, domestic, rib, lean only, roasted - 3 oz.	22.24	69	268	166
Lamb, domestic, shoulder, arm, lean and fat, braised - 3 oz.	25.83	61	260	175
Lamb, domestic, shoulder, arm, lean only, braised - 3 oz.	30.21	65	287	197
Pork and beef sausage, fresh, cooked - 2 links	3.59	209	49	28

Meats:

	Pro	Na	K	P
Pork sausage, fresh, cooked - 2 links	5.11	336	94	48
Pork sausage, fresh, cooked - 1 patty	5.31	349	97	50
Pork bacon, broiled or pan fried - 3 med. slices	5.79	303	92	64
Pork Canadian bacon, grilled - 2 slices	11.27	719	181	138
Pork ham, extra lean, canned, roasted - 3 oz.	17.80	908	298	188
Pork ham, lean and fat, roasted - 3 oz.	18.33	1009	243	182
Pork ham, lean only, roasted - 3 oz.	21.29	1128	269	193
Pork fresh back ribs, lean and fat, roasted - 3 oz.	20.62	86	268	166
Pork fresh leg, lean and fat, roasted - 3 oz.	22.81	51	299	224
Pork fresh leg, lean only, roasted - 3 oz.	25.00	54	317	239

Dialysis Diet

Meats:

	Pro	**Na**	**K**	**P**
Pork loin chops, lean and fat, broiled - 3 oz.	24.40	49	304	197
Pork loin chops, lean and fat, pan fried - 3 oz.	25.42	68	361	220
Pork loin chops, lean only, broiled - 3 oz.	25.66	51	319	205
Pork loin chops, lean only, pan fried - 3 oz.	27.35	73	382	230
Pork loin roast, lean and fat, roasted - 3 oz.	23.30	39	358	196
Pork loin roast, lean only, roasted - 3 oz.	24.41	40	371	201
Pork country style ribs, lean and fat, braised - 3 oz.	20.29	50	279	142
Pork shoulder arm picnic, lean and fat, braised - 3 oz.	23.79	75	314	180
Pork shoulder arm picnic, lean only, braised - 3 oz.	27.42	87	344	192
Pork spareribs, lean and fat, braised - 3 oz.	24.70	79	272	222

Judy Mitzimberg

Meats:

	Pro	Na	K	P
Salami, cooked, beef and pork - 2 slices	7.89	604	112	65
Salami, hard, dry, pork and beef - 2 slices	4.57	372	76	28
Veal, leg (top round), lean and fat, braised - 3 oz.	30.74	57	326	212
Veal, rib, lean and fat, roasted - 3 oz.	20.37	78	251	167
Vienna sausage - 1 sausage	1.65	152	16	8

Miscellaneous Items:

	Pro	Na	K	P
Baking chocolate, unsweetened liquid - 1 oz.	3.43	3	331	96
Baking chocolate, unsweetened squares - 1 square	2.92	4	236	118
Baking powder, double acting - 1 t.	0.00	363	1	101

Dialysis Diet

Miscellaneous Items:

	Pro	Na	K	P
Baking powder, low sodium - 1 t.	0.01	5	505	343
Baking soda - 1 t.	0.00	1259	0	0
Buckwheat flour, whole, groat - 1 c.	15.14	13	692	404
Buckwheat groats, roasted - 1 c.	5.68	7	148	118
Carob flour - 1 T.	0.37	3	6	66
Catsup - 1 packet	0.09	71	2	29
Catsup - 1 T.	0.23	178	6	72
Chives, raw - 1 T.	0.10	0	2	9
Chocolate syrup w/o added nutrients - 1 T.	0.39	14	24	42
Cocoa, dry powder, unsweetened - 1 T.	1.06	1	40	82

Judy Mitzimberg

Miscellaneous Items:

	Pro	**Na**	**K**	**P**
Cornmeal, degermed, enriched, yellow - 1 c.	11.70	4	116	224
Cornmeal, self-rising, degermed, enriched, yellow - 1 c.	11.61	1860	860	235
Cornmeal, whole grain, yellow - 1 c.	9.91	43	294	350
Cornstarch - 1 T.	0.02	1	1	0
Cream of tarter - 1 t.	0.00	2	495	0
Cream substitute, liquid - 1 T.	0.15	12	13	29
Cream substitute, powdered - 1 t.	0.10	4	8	16
Honey, strained or extracted - 1 T.	0.06	1	11	1
Horseradish, prepared - 1 t.	0.06	16	12	2
Hummus, commercial - 1 T.	1.11	53	32	25

Dialysis Diet

Miscellaneous Items:

	Pro	**Na**	**K**	**P**
Jams and preserves - 1 T.	0.07	6	15	2
Jellies - 1 T.	0.04	5	12	1
Lard - 1 T.	0.00	0	0	0
Molasses, black strap - 1 T.	0.00	11	498	8
Mustard, prepared, yellow - 1 t. or packet	0.20	56	8	4
Olives, ripe, canned - 5 large	0.18	192	2	1
Peanut butter, chunk style w/salt - 1 T.	3.85	78	120	51
Peanut butter, smooth style w/salt - 1 T.	4.03	75	107	59
Pickle relish, sweet - 1 T.	0.06	122	4	2
Pickles, cucumber, dill - 1 pickle	0.40	833	75	14

Judy Mitzimberg

Miscellaneous Items:

	Pro	**Na**	**K**	**P**
Seaweed, kelp, raw - 2 T.	0.17	23	9	4
Seaweed, spirulina, dried - 1 T.	0.53	10	13	1
Shortening, soybean, cottonseed - 1 T.	0.00	0	0	0
Sour dressing, non-butterfat, cultured, filled, cream type - 1 T.	0.39	6	19	10
Spices, celery salt - 1 t.	0.36	3	28	11
Spices, chili powder - 1 t.	0.32	26	50	8
Spices, cinnamon, ground - 1 t.	0.09	1	12	1
Spices, curry powder - 1 t.	0.25	1	31	7
Spices, dill weed, fresh - 5 sprigs	0.03	1	7	1

Dialysis Diet

Miscellaneous Items:

	Pro	**Na**	**K**	**P**
Spices, garlic powder - 1 t.	0.47	1	31	12
Spices, onion powder - 1 t.	0.21	1	20	7
Spices, oregano, ground - 1 t.	0.17	0	25	3
Spices, paprika - 1 t.	0.31	1	49	7
Spices, parsley, raw - 10 sprigs	0.30	6	55	6
Spices, pepper, black - 1 t.	0.23	1	26	4
Soy milk, fluid - 1 c.	6.74	29	345	120
Syrup, chocolate - 1 T.	0.87	66	69	26
Syrup, corn, light - 1 T.	0.00	24	1	0
Syrup, maple - 1 T.	0.00	2	41	0

Judy Mitzimberg

Miscellaneous Items:

	Pro	Na	K	P
Syrup, table blend, pancake - 1 T.	0.00	17	0	2
Tapioca, pearl, dry - 1 c.	0.29	2	17	11
Tufu, firm, prepared - 1/4 block	6.51	6	143	119
Tofu, soft, prepared - 1 pc.	7.86	10	144	110
Vanilla extract - 1 t.	0.00	0	6	0
Vegetable oil, canola - 1 T.	0.00	0	0	0
Vinegar, cider - 1 T.	0.00	0	15	1
Wheat flour, all purpose, bleached, enriched - 1 c.	12.91	3	134	135
Wheat flour, all purpose, self-rising, enriched - 1 c.	12.36	1588	155	744
Wheat flour, white, bread, enriched - 1 c.	16.41	3	137	133

Dialysis Diet

Miscellaneous Items:

	Pro	Na	K	P
Wheat flour, cake, enriched - 1 c.	11.23	3	144	116
Wheat flour, whole grain - 1 c.	16.44	6	486	415
Yeast, bakers, active, dry - 1 t.	1.53	2	80	52
Yeast, bakers, active, dry - 1 package	2.68	4	140	90
Yeast, bakers, compressed - 1 cake	1.43	5	102	57

Nuts and Seeds:

	Pro	Na	K	P
Almonds - 1 oz. (24 nuts)	6.03	0	206	134
Brazilnuts, dried, unblanched - 1 oz. (6-8 nuts)	4.07	1	170	170
Cashews, dry roasted w/salt - 1 oz.	4.34	181	160	139

Judy Mitzimberg

Nuts and Seeds:

	Pro	Na	K	P
Cashews, oil roasted w/salt - 1 oz. (18 nuts)	4.58	177	150	121
Chestnuts, European, roasted - 1 c.	4.53	3	847	153
Coconut meat, dried, sweetened, shredded - 1 c.	2.68	244	313	100
Coconut meat, raw - 1 pc.	1.50	9	160	51
Hazelnuts or filberts - 1 oz.	4.24	0	193	82
Macadamias, dry roasted w/salt - (10-12 nuts)	2.21	75	103	56
Mixed nuts, dry roasted w/peanuts - 1 oz.	4.90	190	169	123
Mixed nuts, oil roasted w/peanuts - 1 oz.	4.75	185	165	132
Pecans - 1 oz. (20 halves)	2.60	0	116	79
Pine nuts, pignolia, dried - 1 oz.	6.80	1	170	44

Dialysis Diet

Nuts and Seeds:

	Pro	Na	K	P
Pine nuts, pignolia, dried - 1 T.	2.06	0	52	144
Pistachios, dry roasted w/salt - 1 oz. (47 nuts)	6.05	115	295	137
Walnuts, English - 1 oz. (14 halves)	4.32	1	125	98
Seeds, alfalfa, sprouted, raw - 1 c.	1.32	2	26	23
Seeds, pumpkin and squash, roasted w/salt - 1 oz.	9.35	163	229	332
Seeds, sesame butter, roasted - 1 T.	2.55	17	62	110
Seeds, sesame kernels, dried - 1 T.	2.11	3	33	62
Seeds, sunflower, dry roasted w/salt - 1/4 c.	6.19	250	272	370
Seeds, sunflower, dry roasted w/salt - 1 oz.	5.48	221	241	327

Judy Mitzimberg

Pasta, Rice, and Beans:

	Pro	**Na**	**K**	**P**
Barley, pearled, cooked - 1 c.	3.55	5	146	85
Barley, pearled, raw - 1 c.	19.82	18	560	442
Beans, black, boiled w/o salt - 1 c.	15.24	2	611	241
Beans, great northern, boiled w/o salt - 1 c.	14.74	4	692	292
Beans, kidney, canned - 1 c.	13.44	873	658	241
Beans, kidney, boiled w/o salt - 1 c.	15.35	4	713	251
Beans, navy, boiled w/o salt - 1 c.	15.83	2	670	286
Beans, pinto, boiled w/o salt - 1 c.	14.04	3	800	274
Couscous, cooked - 1 c.	5.95	8	91	35
Couscous, dry - 1 c.	22.07	17	287	294

Dialysis Diet

Pasta, Rice, and Beans:

	Pro	Na	K	P
Lentils, mature seeds, boiled w/o salt - 1 c.	17.86	4	731	356
Macaroni, cooked, enriched - 1 c.	6.68	1	43	76
Noodles, Chinese, chow mein - 1 c.	3.77	198	54	72
Noodles, egg, cooked, enriched - 1 c.	7.60	11	45	110
Noodles, egg, spinach, cooked, enriched - 1 c.	8.06	19	59	91
Rice, brown, long-grain, cooked - 1 c.	5.03	10	84	162
Rice, white, long-grain, parboiled - 1 c.	4.01	5	65	74
Rice, white, long-grain, dry, enriched - 1 c.	12.56	9	222	252
Rice, white, long-grain, pre-cooked or instant, enriched, prepared - 1 c.	3.40	5	7	23

Judy Mitzimberg

Pasta, Rice, and Beans:

	Pro	Na	K	P
Rice, white, long-grain, regular, cooked - 1 c.	4.25	2	55	68
Rice, white, long-grain, regular, raw - 1 c.	13.19	9	213	213
Spaghetti, cooked w/o salt - 1 c.	6.68	1	43	76
Spaghetti, whole wheat, cooked - 1 c.	7.46	4	62	125
Wild rice, cooked - 1 c.	6.54	5	166	134

Poultry:

	Pro	Na	K	P
Chicken roll, light meat - 2 slices	11.07	331	129	89
Chicken breast w/skin, batter fried - 1/2 breast	34.78	385	281	259
Chicken breast w/skin, fried w/flour - 1/2 breast	31.20	75	254	228

Dialysis Diet

Poultry:

	Pro	Na	K	P
Chicken breast w/o skin, roasted - 1/2 breast	26.68	64	220	196
Chicken, dark meat w/o skin, fried - 3 oz.	24.35	81	213	157
Chicken drumstick w/skin, batter fried - 1	15.80	194	134	106
Chicken drumstick w/skin, fried w/flour - 1	13.21	44	112	86
Chicken drumstick w/o skin, roasted - 1	12.45	42	108	81
Chicken giblets, simmered - 1 c.	34.48	84	229	332
Chicken, light meat w/o skin, fried - 3 oz.	27.57	68	221	194
Chicken neck w/o skin, simmered - 1 neck	4.42	12	25	23
Chicken thigh w/skin, batter fried - 1	18.58	248	165	133
Chicken thigh w/o skin, roasted - 1	13.49	46	124	95

Judy Mitzimberg

Poultry:

	Pro	Na	K	P
Chicken wing w/skin, batter fried - 1	9.74	157	68	59
Chicken, canned w/broth - 5 oz.	30.91	714	196	158
Chicken liver, simmered - 1 liver	4.77	10	27	61
Chicken stewing, stewed - 1 c.	42.59	109	283	286
Duck, domesticated w/o skin, roasted - 1/2 duck	51.89	144	557	449
Turkey patties, breaded, fried - 1 patty	8.96	512	176	173
Turkey roast, boneless, frozen, roasted - 3 oz.	18.13	578	253	208
Turkey, dark meat, roasted - 3 oz.	24.00	66	244	171
Turkey giblets, simmered - 1 c.	38.53	86	290	296
Turkey, ground, cooked - 1 patty	22.44	88	221	161

Dialysis Diet

Poultry:

	Pro	Na	K	P
Turkey, light meat, roasted - 3 oz.	25.12	54	256	184
Turkey, meat only, roasted - 1 c.	41.05	98	417	298
Turkey neck, simmered - 1 neck	40.80	85	226	185

Salad Dressings:

	Pro	Na	K	P
Blue or roquefort cheese, commercial w/salt - 1 T.	0.73	167	6	11
French, commercial w/salt - 1 T.	0.09	214	12	3
French, low-fat w/salt - 1 T.	0.03	128	13	2
French, homemade - 1 T.	0.01	92	3	0

Judy Mitzimberg

Salad Dressings:

	Pro	Na	K	P
Home recipe, cooked - 1 T.	0.67	117	19	14
Home recipe, vinegar and oil - 1 T.	0.00	0	1	0
Italian, commercial, low-cal w/salt - 1 T.	0.02	118	2	1
Italian, commercial, regular - 1 T.	0.10	116	2	1
Mayonnaise, soybean oil w/salt - 1 T.	0.15	78	5	4
Russian, low-cal w/salt - 1 T.	0.08	141	26	6
Russian, regular w/salt - 1 T.	0.24	133	24	6
Thousand Island, commercial, regular - 1 T.	0.14	109	18	3
Thousand Island, low-cal w/salt - 1 T.	0.12	153	17	3

Dialysis Diet

Sauces and Gravies:

	Pro	Na	K	P
Barbeque sauce - 1 T.	0.28	128	27	3
Cheese sauce, ready-to-serve - 1/4 c.	4.23	522	19	99
Homemade white, medium - 1 c.	9.60	885	390	245
Pasta, spaghetti/marinar, ready-to-serve - 1 c.	3.55	1030	738	80
Pepper, ready-to-serve - 1 T.	0.02	124	7	1
Salsa - 1 T.	0.20	69	34	4
Soy sauce - 1 T.	0.83	914	29	18
Teriyaki - 1 T.	1.07	690	41	28
Tomato sauce, canned - 1 c.	3.26	1482	909	78

Judy Mitzimberg

	Pro	**Na**	**K**	**P**
Beef gravy, canned - 1/4 c.	2.18	326	47	17
Country sausage gravy, ready-to-serve - 1/4 c.	2.85	236	48	25
Mushroom gravy, canned - 1/4 c.	0.75	340	63	9
Turkey gravy, canned - 1/4 c.	1.55	344	65	17

Snacks:

	Pro	Na	K	P
Beef jerkey, chopped and formed - 1 lg. pc.	6.57	438	118	81
Chex mix - 2/3 c.	3.12	288	76	53
Corn-based chips, plain - 1 oz.	1.87	179	40	52
Corn-based puffs or twists, cheese flavored - 1 oz.	2.15	298	47	31

Dialysis Diet

Snacks:

	Pro	Na	K	P
Fruit leather rolls - 1 lg.	0.21	13	62	7
Granola bars, hard, plain - 1 bar	2.86	83	95	79
Granola bars, soft, coated - 1 bar	2.89	55	96	64
Granola bars, soft, uncoated, chocolate chip - 1 bar	2.07	77	96	65
Granola bars, soft, uncoated, raisin - 1 bar	2.15	80	103	62
Kellogg Nutri Grain cereal bar, fruit - 1 bar	1.63	110	73	38
Kellogg Rice Krispie Treat - 1 bar	0.75	77	9	9
Oriental mix, rice based - 1/4 c.	4.91	117	93	74
Popcorn, air popped - 1 c.	0.96	0	24	24
Popcorn cakes - 1 cake	0.97	29	33	28

Judy Mitzimberg

Snacks:

	Pro	Na	K	P
Popcorn, caramel coated w/peanuts - 1 c.	2.69	124	149	53
Popcorn, cheese flavored - 1 c.	1.02	98	29	40
Popcorn, oil popped - 1 c.	0.99	97	25	28
Pork skins, plain - 1 oz.	17.38	521	36	24
Potato chips, plain, salted - 1 oz.	1.98	168	361	47
Potato chips, plain, unsalted - 1 oz.	1.98	2	361	47
Potato chips, sour cream and onion - 1 oz.	2.30	177	377	50
Pretzels, hard, plain, salted - 10	5.46	1029	88	6
Tortilla chips, plain - 1 oz.	1.98	150	56	58
Trail mix, regular - 1 c.	20.37	177	946	565

Dialysis Diet

Soups:

	Pro	Na	K	P
Bean w/ham, ready-to-serve - 1 c.	12.61	972	425	143
Bean w/pork, prepared w/water - 1 c.	7.89	951	402	132
Beef broth, bouillon, consomme, prepared w/water	5.35	636	154	31
Beef noodle, prepared w/water - 1 c.	4.83	952	100	46
Chicken noodle, ready-to-serve - 1 c.	12.72	850	108	72
Chicken noodle, prepared w/water - 1 c.	4.05	1106	55	36
Chicken noodle, dehydrated, prepared w/water - 1 c.	2.12	578	33	30
Chicken w/rice, prepared w/water - 1 c.	3.54	815	101	22
Clam chowder, Manhattan style, prepared w/water - 1 c.	2.20	578	188	41
Clam chowder, New England style, prepared w/milk - 1 c.	9.47	992	300	156

Judy Mitzimberg

Soups:

	Pro	Na	K	P
Cream of mushroom, prepared w/milk - 1 c.	6.05	918	270	156
Cream of mushroom, prepared w/water - 1 c.	2.32	881	100	49
Minestrone, prepared w/water - 1 c.	4.27	911	313	55
Onion, dehydrated, prepared w/water - 1 c.	1.11	849	64	30
Pea, green, prepared w/water - 1 c.	8.60	918	190	125
Soup stock, fish, homemade - 1 c.	5.27	363	336	130
Tomato, prepared w/milk - 1 c.	6.10	744	449	149
Tomato, prepared w/water - 1 c.	2.05	695	264	.34
Vegetable beef prepared w/water - 1 c.	5.59	791	173	41
Vegetarian vegetable prepared w/water - 1 c.	2.10	822	210	34

Dialysis Diet

Soups:
Progresso Brand Healthy Classics:

	Pro	**Na**	**K**	**P**
Chicken noodle - 1 c.	5.74	460	209	85
Chicken rice w/vegetables - 1 c.	6.26	459	275	88
Lentil - 1 c.	7.79	443	336	128
Ministrone - 1 c.	4.77	470	306	87
New England clam chowder - 1 c.	5.20	529	283	59
Vegetable - 1 c.	4.19	466	290	74

Note: These soups have a lower content of sodium but are still higher than recipes made from scratch.

Vegetables:

	Pro	Na	K	P
Artichokes, boiled w/o salt - 1 c.	5.85	160	595	144
Artichokes, boiled w/o salt - 1 med.	4.18	114	425	103
Asparagus, canned, drained - 4 spears	1.54	207	124	31
Asparagus, fresh, boiled, drained - 4 spears	1.55	7	96	32
Asparagus, frozen, boiled w/o salt - 1 c.	5.31	7	392	99
Asparagus, frozen, boiled w/o salt - 4 spears	1.77	2	131	33
Bamboo shoots, canned, drained - 1 c.	2.25	9	105	33
Beans, baked, canned - 1 c.	12.17	1008	752	264
Beans, baked w/franks - 1 c.	17.48	1114	609	269
Beans, green, canned - 1 c.	1.55	354	147	26

Dialysis Diet

Vegetables:

	Pro	**Na**	**K**	**P**
Beans, green, fresh, boiled w/o salt - 1 c.	2.36	4	374	49
Beans, green, frozen, boiled w/o salt - 1 c.	2.01	12	170	42
Beans, white, canned - 1 c.	19.02	13	1189	238
Beets, canned - 1 beet	0.22	4	36	47
Beets, canned - 1 c.	1.55	29	252	330
Beets, fresh, boiled w/o salt - 1 c.	2.86	65	519	131
Beets, fresh, boiled w/o salt - 1 beet	0.84	19	153	39
Broccoli, fresh, boiled w/o salt - 1 spear	1.10	10	108	22
Broccoli, fresh, boiled w/o salt - 1 c.	4.65	41	456	92
Broccoli, flower cluster, raw - 1 floweret	0.33	3	36	7

Judy Mitzimberg

Vegetables:

	Pro	Na	K	P
Broccoli, frozen, boiled w/o salt - 1 c.	5.70	44	331	101
Broccoli, raw - 1 c.	2.62	24	286	58
Brussel sprouts, fresh, boiled w/o salt - 1 c.	3.98	33	495	87
Brussel sprouts, frozen, boiled w/o salt - 1 c.	5.64	36	504	84
Cabbage, Chinese (pak-choi), boiled w/o salt - 1 c.	2.65	58	631	49
Cabbage, Chinese (pe-tsai), boiled w/o salt - 1 c.	1.79	11	268	46
Cabbage, fresh, boiled w/o salt - 1 c.	1.53	12	146	23
Cabbage, raw - 1 c.	1.01	13	172	16
Cabbage, red, raw - 1 c.	0.97	8	144	29
Carrots, baby, raw - 1 med.	0.08	4	28	4

Dialysis Diet

Vegetables:

	Pro	Na	K	P
Carrots, canned - 1 c.	0.93	333	261	35
Carrots, fresh, boiled w/o salt - 1 c.	1.70	103	354	47
Carrots, frozen, boiled w/o salt - 1 c.	1.74	86	231	38
Carrots, raw - 1 c.	1.13	39	355	48
Cauliflower, fresh, boiled w/o salt - 1 c.	2.28	19	176	40
Cauliflower, fresh, boiled w/o salt - 3 flowerets	0.99	8	77	17
Cauliflower, frozen, boiled w/o salt - 1 c.	2.90	32	250	43
Cauliflower, raw - 1 c.	1.98	30	303	44
Cauliflower, raw - 1 floweret	0.26	4	39	6
Celery, fresh, boiled w/o salt - 1 c.	1.25	137	426	38

Judy Mitzimberg

Vegetables:

	Pro	Na	K	P
Celery, raw - 1 c.	0.90	104	344	30
Celery, raw - 1 stalk	0.30	35	115	10
Chickpeas (garbanzo beans), canned - 1 c.	11.88	718	413	216
Chickpeas, fresh, boiled w/o salt - 1 c.	14.53	11	477	276
Coleslaw, homemade - 1 c.	1.55	28	217	38
Collards, fresh, boiled w/o salt - 1 c.	4.01	17	494	49
Collards, frozen, boiled w/o salt - 1 c.	5.05	85	427	46
Corn, sweet, white, boiled w/o salt - 1 ear	2.56	13	192	79
Corn, yellow, canned cream style - 1 c.	4.45	730	343	131
Corn, yellow, canned vacuum pack - 1 c.	5.06	571	391	134

Dialysis Diet

Vegetables:

	Pro	**Na**	**K**	**P**
Corn, yellow, fresh, boiled w/o salt - 1 ear	2.56	13	192	79
Corn, yellow, frozen, boiled w/o salt - 1 c.	4.51	8	241	93
Corn, yellow, frozen, boiled w/o salt - 1 ear	1.96	3	158	47
Cucumber, peeled, raw - 1 lg.	1.60	6	414	25
Cucumber, peeled, raw - 1 c.	0.68	2	176	59
Dandelion greens, fresh, boiled w/o salt - 1 c.	2.10	46	244	44
Eggplant, fresh, boiled w/o salt - 1 c.	0.82	3	246	22
Endive, raw - 1 c.	0.63	11	157	14
Garlic, raw - 1 clove	0.19	1	12	5
Hearts of palm, canned - 1 pc.	0.83	141	58	21

Judy Mitzimberg

Vegetables:

	Pro	Na	K	P
Jerusalem artichokes, raw - 1 c.	3.00	6	644	117
Kale, fresh, boiled w/o salt - 1 c.	2.47	30	296	36
Kale, frozen, boiled w/o salt - 1 c.	3.69	20	417	36
Kohlrabi, fresh, boiled w/o salt - 1 c.	2.97	35	561	74
Leeks, fresh, boiled w/o salt - 1 c.	0.84	10	90	18
Lentils, boiled w/o salt - 1 c.	17.86	4	731	356
Lettuce, raw - 1 med. leaf	0.10	0	19	2
Lettuce, raw - 1 head	2.10	8	419	37
Parsnips, fresh, boiled w/o salt - 1 c.	2.06	16	573	108
Peas, fresh, podded, boiled w/o salt - 1 c.	5.23	6	384	88

Dialysis Diet

Vegetables:

	Pro	Na	K	P
Peas, frozen, boiled w/o salt - 1 c.	5.60	8	347	93
Peas, green, canned - 1 c.	7.51	428	294	114
Peas, split, boiled w/o salt - 1 c.	16.35	4	710	194
Peppers, hot chili, green, raw - 1 pepper	0.90	3	153	21
Peppers, hot chili, red, raw - 1 pepper	0.90	3	153	21
Peppers, jalapeno, canned - 1/4 c.	0.24	434	50	5
Peppers, sweet, green, boiled w/o salt - 1 c.	1.25	3	226	24
Peppers, sweet, green, raw - 1 ring	0.09	0	18	2
Peppers, sweet, green, raw - 1 pepper	1.06	2	211	23
Peppers, sweet, green, raw - 1 c.	1.33	3	264	28

Vegetables:

	Pro	Na	K	P
Peppers, sweet, red, boiled w/o salt - 1 c.	1.25	3	226	24
Peppers, sweet, red, raw - 1 c.	1.33	3	264	28
Peppers, sweet, red, raw - 1 pepper	1.06	2	211	2
Pimento, canned - 1 T.	0.13	2	19	2
Potato pancakes, homemade - 1	4.68	386	597	84
Potato salad, homemade - 1 c.	6.70	1323	635	130
Potatoes au gratin, dry mix, prepared - 1 c.	5.64	1076	537	233
Potatoes au gratin, homemade - 1 c.	12.40	1061	970	277
Potato, baked w/skin - 1	4.65	16	844	115
Potato, baked w/o skin - 1	3.06	8	610	78

Dialysis Diet

Vegetables:

	Pro	Na	K	P
Potato skins, baked w/o salt - 1 skin	2.49	12	332	59
Potato, boiled w/skin, w/o salt - 1	2.54	5	515	60
Potato, boiled w/o skin, w/o salt - 1 c.	2.67	8	512	62
Potatoes, French fried, homemade, w/o salt, heated in oven - 10 fries	1.59	15	209	41
Potatoes, frozen, hash browns - 1 patty	0.92	10	126	21
Potatoes, hash brown, homemade - 1 c.	3.78	37	501	66
Potatoes, mashed, from flakes, w/whole milk and butter - 1 c.	3.99	697	489	118
Potatoes, mashed, homemade - 1 c.	4.07	636	628	101

Judy Mitzimberg

Vegetables:

	Pro	Na	K	P
Potatoes, scalloped, dry mix, prepared - 1 c.	5.19	835	497	137
Potatoes, scalloped, homemade w/butter - 1 c.	7.03	821	926	154
Pumpkin, canned w/o salt - 1 c.	2.70	12	505	86
Pumpkin, boiled w/o salt - 1 c.	1.76	2	564	74
Radishes, raw - 1 radish	0.03	1	10	1
Refried beans, canned - 1 c.	13.83	753	673	217
Rutabagas, fresh, boiled w/o salt - 1 c.	2.19	34	554	95
Sauerkraut, canned - 1 c.	2.15	1560	401	47
Shallots, raw - 1 T.	0.25	1	33	6
Soybeans, green, boiled w/o salt - 1 c.	22.23	25	970	284

Dialysis Diet

Vegetables:

	Pro	Na	K	P
Soybeans, mature, boiled w/o salt - 1 c.	28.62	2	886	421
Spinach, canned - 1 c.	6.01	58	740	94
Spinach, fresh, boiled w/o salt - 1 c.	5.35	126	839	101
Spinach, frozen, boiled w/o salt - 1 c.	5.97	163	566	91
Spinach, raw - 1 leaf	0.29	8	56	5
Spinach, raw - 1 c.	0.86	24	167	15
Squash, summer, boiled w/o salt - 1 c.	1.64	2	346	70
Squash, summer, raw - 1 c.	1.33	2	220	40
Squash, winter, baked w/o salt - 1 c.	1.82	2	869	41
Squash, winter, frozen, boiled w/o salt - 1 c.	2.95	5	319	34

Judy Mitzimberg

Vegetables:

	Pro	Na	K	P
Sweet potato, canned, syrup pack - 1 c.	2.51	76	378	49
Sweet, potato, canned, vacuum pack - 1 c.	4.21	135	796	125
Sweet potato, baked in skin - 1	2.51	15	508	80
Sweet potato, boiled w/o skin - 1	2.57	20	287	42
Sweet potato, candied, homemade - 1 pc.	0.91	74	198	27
Tomatillos, raw - 1 med.	0.33	0	91	13
Tomatoes, canned, stewed - 1 c.	2.42	564	607	51
Tomatoes, canned, whole - 1 c.	2.21	355	530	46
Tomatoes, red, ripe, raw - 1 cherry tomato	0.14	2	38	4
Tomatoes, red, ripe, raw - 1 slice	0.17	2	44	5

Dialysis Diet

Vegetables:

	Pro	Na	K	P
Tomatoes, red, ripe, raw - 1 tomato	1.05	11	273	30
Tomatoes, sun-dried - 1 pc.	0.28	42	69	7
Tomatoes, sun-dried, oil packed - 1 pc.	0.15	8	47	4
Turnip greens, fresh, boiled w/o salt - 1 c.	1.64	42	292	42
Turnips, fresh, boiled w/o salt - 1 c.	1.11	78	211	30
Turnip greens, frozen, boiled w/o salt - 1 c.	5.49	25	367	56
Vegetables, mixed, canned - 1 c.	4.22	243	474	68
Vegetables, mixed, frozen, boiled w/o salt - 1 c.	5.21	64	308	93
Water chestnuts, Chinese, canned - 1 c.	1.23	11	165	27

Judy Mitzimberg

Resources

There are many wonderful web sites that you can visit to obtain additional information about hemodialysis and the renal diet. Below I have listed a few:

National Kidney Foundation
www.kidney.com

National Institute of Diabetes and Digestive and Kidney Disease
www.niddk.nih.gov

Combined Health Information Database
www.chid.nih.gov

Worldwide Kidney Disease Community
www.ikidney.com

Nephron Information Center
www.nephron.com

American Kidney Fund
www.aakp.org

Kidney and Urology Foundation of America
www.kidneyurology.org

RenalWeb
www.renalweb.com

There are also some excellent resources for sample menus:

www.kidneyschool.org This site offers a free two week cycle of menus from the Living Well cookbook which is free to patients from Amgen.

There is a book called *Magic Menus* which is available from NKF of North Texas. This can be obtained by calling 214-351-2392.

There are several other good references for patients on the **iKidney.com** website.

ORDER FORM

Fill out the order form below and mail with a check or credit card information to:

ADL Publishing
P.O. Box 2791
Glendale, AZ 85311-2791
Ph: 623-842-9123

Name_____

Address_____

City, State & Zip_____

$16.95 + $3.85 priority shipping

Check Enclosed ☐

Credit Card ☐

Card Number_____

Expiration Date_____

Signature_____

Refund Policy:
We guarantee your satisfaction. Order this book and look it over. You may return it within 30 days if not fully satisfied and your full purchase price will be refunded, no questions asked.

ORDER FORM

Fill out the order form below and mail with a check or credit card information to:

**ADL Publishing
P.O. Box 2791
Glendale, AZ 85311-2791
Ph: 623-842-9123**

Name_____

Address_____

City, State & Zip_____

$16.95 + $3.85 priority shipping

Check Enclosed ☐

Credit Card ☐

Card Number_____

Expiration Date_____

Signature_____

Refund Policy:
We guarantee your satisfaction. Order this book and look it over. You may return it within 30 days if not fully satisfied and your full purchase price will be refunded, no questions asked.

NOTES